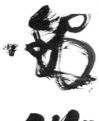

"I have known Dr. Hin and watched him at work for so long now. His technical skill goes hand in hand with that same wisdom, generosity and spiritual strength that have now found expression in his book. I am sure that the reader will find there not only valuable information and advice concerning disorders from which one may suffer and be healed, but likewise a great medicine that is not available even on prescription: serenity, a quiet mind."—Professor Jacques Panijel, C.N.R.S., Paris.

DR KUAN HIN
CHINESE MASSAGE AND ACUPRESSURE

ENGLISH VERSION BY
NANCY DARGEL

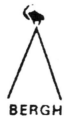

BERGH

BERGH PUBLISHING, Inc.
276 Fifth Avenue, New York, N.Y. 10001

CONTENTS

Introducing Dr. Kuan Hin	7
Inhoa	11
Introduction to Chinese medicine	19
The practice of Chinese medicine	29
The Eight Wonders of Chinese massage	43
Acupressure: healing with the hands	71
Nervosity	107
Palpitations	111
Depression	115
Insomnia	119
Headache	125
Debility	133
Vertigo	137
How to stop smoking	141
Pain	145
Digestion	165
The respiratory tract	179
Urogenital disorders	189
Skin diseases	203
Varicose veins	209
Inflammation of the eyes	213
High blood pressure	217
Medical co-operation between East and West	221
Glossary	227

This type of drawing requires energy, inspiration and peace of mind. It takes only a moment to put it onto paper, but every stroke of the brush is a symbol, not one was drawn by chance.

INTRODUCING DR KUAN HIN

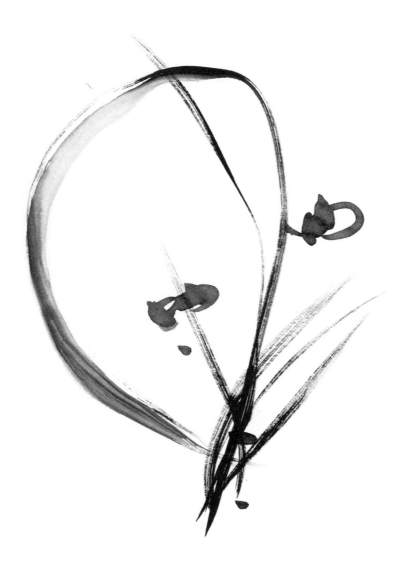

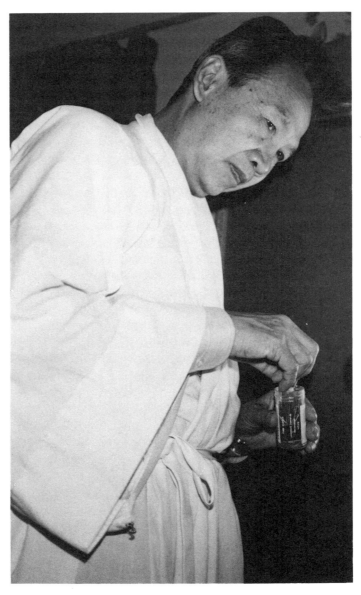

Dr. Kuan Hin in preparation. Every treatment demands maximum concentration and serenity.

Ever since we were air-borne at Zurich, I had been surreptitiously watching the Oriental gentleman in the next seat. He had a kindly look; his short-cropped hair was very black; I wondered how old he was—might be forty, or fifty, perhaps more. His hands, playing with the lock of the brief-case on his knee, were long and slender with carefully trimmed nails. Suddenly, he snapped his case open and inside it I saw row upon row of what could only be hyperdermic needles, obviously belonging to a syringe—he must be a fixer! or else an addict! He had heard me gasp and he looked around quickly, without closing his case . . .

By the time we landed at Orly, I had learnt a little about acupuncture and my headache had been cured by acupressure, a therapy technique of which I had not previously heard the name.

That was my first, chance meeting with Dr. Hin. Since then I have become one of his regular patients and consult him whenever I am in Paris. The following brief outline of his life-story is my contribution to this book.

Dr. Kuan Hin was born in Canton on January 22nd, in 1922, a year that was under the sign of the Dog. His natural environment was the world of medicine; his mother, like many women in the family before her, was a physician. When still a very small boy, Kuan was allowed to watch her at work and soon to extract the acupuncture needles when a treatment was completed. He was found to have "healing hands"; he could join in the collecting and drying of herbs for the preparation of medicine. Kuan's father was in business and the family moved to Haiphong when the child was five, then on to Yüennen, some ten years later. It was a restless period, but there were no interruptions in Kuan's own schooling and medical training. He completed his studies at the University of Shang-Hai in the Tong-Nann Faculty of Medicine and was mobilized in the Army Medical Corps. China was at war with Japan from 1931 to 1945. Viet-Nam proclaimed its independence in 1945 and found itself at war with France. Dr. Hin, by then an army surgeon with field rank, was put in charge of the Potchi military hospital at Hanoi. There, his physician's vocation to save human lives without regard for creed or color at length jeopardised his personal security and he made his way to Europe, where he first found employment with a business-firm in Paris and then gradually established contact with Western medical men, offering them his Oriental techniques and practice in support of their own. People discovered that the "Chinese doctor" could relieve pain; he cured their migraine; he restored mobility to musicians' fingers, as well as to the limbs of children who had been crippled from birth; he cured cases of Cancer. Dr. Kuan Hin is now a physician of international repute. He still staggers his fees according to the patient's means, as he used to do in his first practice in the *XI° arrondissement,* where his wife and two of his eight children still operate. There are two hospitals for crippled children under his personal supervision in Denmark. At the present time he is throwing the full strength of his knowledge and skill into the fight against AIDS.

The image of Dr. Hin in Oriental robes, surrounded with acupuncture needles and grateful letters from his patients, cannot be disconnected from that of the Parisian Consultant, working in close co-operation with his Western colleagues, convinced that the two schools of medicine are usefully complementary, nor yet finally from that of the spiritual adept, humbly sharing with his fellow-men time-proven knowledge of our bodies and how to tend and heal them, lessons of positive approach to each day's burden of good or ill, and of that self-discipline no-one of us may cease from learning until our life's end.

(from the story of Dr. Hin as told by Verena Bürki)

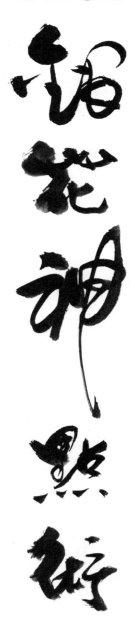

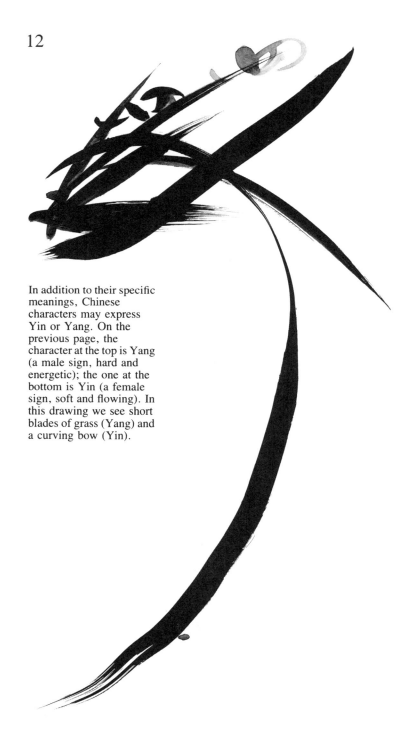

In addition to their specific meanings, Chinese characters may express Yin or Yang. On the previous page, the character at the top is Yang (a male sign, hard and energetic); the one at the bottom is Yin (a female sign, soft and flowing). In this drawing we see short blades of grass (Yang) and a curving bow (Yin).

A senior Army Officer, a retired General, once came to me with a personal problem: as soon as he heard military music—usually when attending some commemorative ceremony in an official capacity and in uniform—tears would fill his eyes and start streaming down his face. The phenomenon was entirely beyond his control. On the following such occasion, just before he went in to take his stand, I inserted an acupuncture needle at a chosen point in his wrist and left it there. The band played and the old soldier took the salute, calmly and unmoved. I cannot say whether it was the presence of the needle or his knowledge of it that worked the cure, but both without doubt were equally necessary.

I have recorded the story of the *Weeping General* at the beginning of this book, because it illustrates a principle that is valid in every sphere of preventive medicine. Mind and body are integral components of the same entity and their interaction can be positive or negative in effect. The success of a treatment, be it preventive or curative, is best ensured when the patient has confidence not only in the treatment but also in himself. This requires equanimity and strength of mind. The proposals for therapy contained in this book seek not only to maintain or restore the body's health, but also to strengthen the spirit. As you will see, this is often achieved by the concrete means of acupressure, a pressure exerted on specific points of the anatomy. Mind and body are linked in a network of energy relationships that react with extreme sensitivity even to the gentle touch of a finger. Chinese medicine is built up on this fact as on its very foundation and therefore so too is Inhoa, a method issued from one of China's oldest medical schools.

Prior to further discussion of Chinese medicine and the practical applications of Inhoa, I should perhaps explain what Inhoa actually is. How does it work? What diseases can be cured by this method? Can it be mis-applied? Are there counter-indications?

What Is Inhoa?

Inhoa means *silver flower*. It was the name that our ancestors gave to their method of preventing or healing in ages past and that has been handed down, enriched by new knowledge, from generation to generation. When I speak of my own ancestors I must use the feminine form of the noun, for it was from mother to daughter that the Inhoa tradition was handed down in our family. Avowedly, this is contrary to custom and there has certainly been no attempt to dissuade the males from entering the profession. Yet I am still the exception: my sister maintains and develops Inhoa at home in Canton and among my own children it is my daughter, Cok Kan, who has gone deepest into the method here. Inhoa rejects no means that may preserve or restore health. We work with all the Chinese techniques available to us and offer whatever knowledge we possess in co-operation with school medicine and alternative medicine of the Western world. Our main fields are acupuncture, acupressure and massage, and likewise dietetics, herbal therapy and yoga. This book concerns itself solely with Chinese massage and acupressure, both of which are ideal areas for an introduction to self-treatment, since they demand of the trainee only rudimentary knowledge and no kind of equipment. It will be with his bare hands, stimulating the energy flows of the body, that he may work miracles. Inhoa can indeed prove miraculous in its effects. It is like the final drop of water that makes the ocean overflow, or the pressure of a child's hand applied at a certain point, that can set a heavy truck in motion after the joint efforts of several strong men have failed. Simple stimulation by acupuncture may solve problems that appeared to be beyond our ken. I was once consulted by a Danish lady, whose lower limbs had been left paralysed after a surgical operation. At the end of three days intensive treatment, we had her on her feet again. Time has since shown that the cure is of a lasting nature. But whether it should be considered to have been due to chance, or a miracle, or the result of acupuncture, I am quite sure that my own part in it was no more than the ''touch of a child's hand,'' finalizing the work done by my Danish colleagues before me. Inhoa is a gentle method, and while this term is commonly applied to Chinese medicine in general, it is a particularly appropriate one for Inhoa acupressure and massage. If *stroking,* or *fondling,* were medical terms and as clearly defined as the word *massage,* these might be useful substitutes to describe a method where the hand glides over the skin like flowing water. Certain forms of massage are indeed called a *dry bath.* In acupressure, the finger-tips exert rather more pressure, but not enough to require much force. The effect on the energy flow is likewise less direct and less ''forceful'' than that produced by an acupuncture needle. For this very reason, the Inhoa method of massage and acupressure is useful in cases where acupuncture is not advisable for the patient. We frequently observe the beneficial, restorative effect of Inhoa massage on persons who are seriously ill and in a weakened condition. It is like offering a bowl of rice to a starving man; it can mean life itself to him, whereas his well-fed neighbor might set it aside as being of little value.

What Can Inhoa Do?

We have already referred to the significance of energy flows in the body. Energy nourishes the organism, it is life's fuel. It flows through the body, through its every part and one can easily understand the trouble arising from any delay in its supply. Frequently the damage done is not merely local, for the smallest stoppage inevitably leads to a general energy imbalance and can set off disorders in parts of the body not apparently involved. Diseases then lead to further blocking of the energy flow, the immunity system grows weaker and weaker, one may be confronted with an avalanche of multiple symptoms. Obviously prevention is essential!

Prevention is the very core of Chinese medicine. Its dual aim is to preserve the health of the healthy by preventive measures and to restore the health of the sick by curative ones that seek to overcome an existing disease whilst strengthening the body to ward off possible sequellae. Meeting both these demands, Inhoa has always been and remains the precise solution of the problem set us.

If you include *massage* in your daily hygiene, you are making sure of a free flow of energy and will be able to dissipate any obstruction in its earliest stages. This is because the relatively broad surface of your flat hand enables you to massage the whole of your body, thus activating in a short space of time all its meridians, the lines of force that carry energy through the system. Applied to the entire body surface, massage can likewise be used therapeutically; it acts on disorders of the circulation, muscular diseases and inflammation of the joints. Again and again it has worked wonders in nervous conditions due to stress and has proved of inestimable value to persons having to cope with an excessive work-load. A short break, an interval between two appointments, is long enough for a massage and, after taking your mind off your work during the time you are concentrating on massage, the swift, effective action of this relaxation technique will enable you to return to the job perfectly fit and ready to concentrate on that. Full information on each individual massage and its preventive and therapeutic specificity is given in the chapter entitled *The eight wonders of Chinese massage.*

Acupressure is used particularly in acute or chronic conditions and in cases where a disease has already set in. This is inherent in the actual technique, where it is no longer the hand that massages the body, but the finger-tips that exert pressure on well-defined strategic points (acupoints) of the body's surface and by this means activate the meridians. The acupoints are selected according to identical principles in acupuncture and acupressure and are necessarily the same whether they are to be treated with needles or with the finger-tips.

We apply acupressure to points which act directly on an existing symptom and always at the same time on others which have a preventive action as regards possible sequellae of the illness. Further acupoints strengthen the mind and body generally, making the patient better able to stand up to his illness and also to its treatment. Acupressure is eminently appropriate for the treatment of painful motory diseases, headache, digestive and urogenital complaints, as it is too for any kind of neurosis, sleeplessness, addictions, depression. it is most valuable for the long-term treatment of chronic algesic conditions, since the problems connected with the side-effects due to continued use of analgesics do not arise. The simplicity of the technique recommends it for personal use in every-day complaints such as indigestion or the common cold. In China, small children are shown where to press their skin when different things are the matter with them. Finally, acupressure has the advantage of being entirely safe, as long as one observes minimum rules of hygiene and washes one's hands before practising acupressure.

INTRODUCTION TO CHINESE MEDICINE

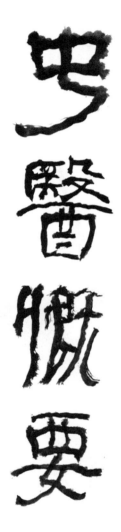

20

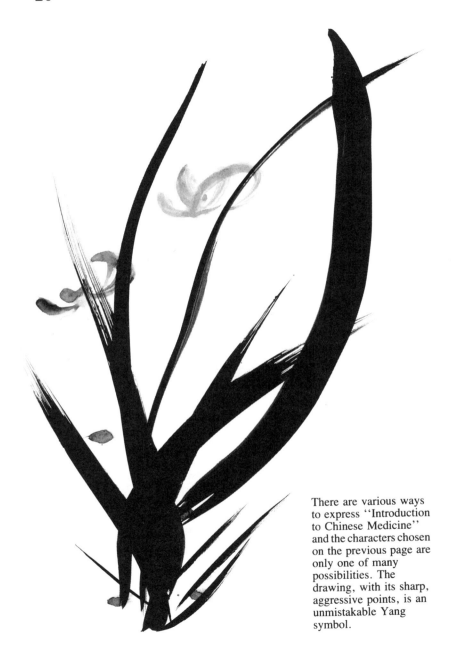

There are various ways
to express ''Introduction
to Chinese Medicine''
and the characters chosen
on the previous page are
only one of many
possibilities. The
drawing, with its sharp,
aggressive points, is an
unmistakable Yang
symbol.

According to the principles of Chinese medicine, a healthy body is a sign of harmonious balance of the Yin and Yang forces flowing through it. Therefore any form of disease is a symptom of energy imbalance.

Historical Background

The knowledge that massage not only relieves pain in given parts of the body, but also produces rapid improvement of its general condition, dates from prehistoric times. The sharpened tools of the Stone Age were used to tend the body as much as for the day's work. The stone artefacts were the first *needles* of acupuncture. The ability to light a fire and the discovery that certain pains were relieved by its warmth, led to the development of *moxibustion,* the second pillar of Chinese medicine, the practice of applying to certain points of the patient's body the heat of burnt and glowing vegetable matter.

The working tools and the acupuncture needles of Ancient China then developed side by side. The sharpened stone was followed by needles of bone and bamboo and the first metal needles appeared in the latter half of the second millenium B.C. Knowledge of the mysterious relationship between the points of insertion and the healing effect produced increased. The system of the meridians and their courses was discovered. The *Huangdi Nei Jing,* the oldest Classic of Chinese Medicine, recorded the state of the art over two thousand years ago. The book contains detailed Minutes of the conversations between the Emperor Huangdi and his physician. Whole sections are devoted to acupuncture, the position, function and disorders of the meridians, the indications and counter-indications concerning the points of insertion.

Localising these puncture points remained a problem for centuries. Patients might be fat or thin, tall or short. Where was the yardstick to provide accurate measurement, since it could not be based on standard units or distance from one point to another? The matter was left largely to the operator's intuition. Under the Han Dynasty (202 B.C.-220 A.D.), a solution was found by taking a relative physical measurement, *Cun* (Tchun) as the unit of measurement. The breadth of the individual patient's thumb becomes the yardstick whereby the position of the acupoints is calculated. *Cun* has continued to be used by practicioners to this day.

Under the Tang Dynasty (618–907), a Chair for Acupuncture and Moxibustion was created at the Chinese universities. The subject was made compulsory for students of medicine. Towards the turn of the century two life-size bronze statues were set up, on which the teachers had marked the course of the meridians and the position of the acupoints, and these became the basic textbook for training and final examinations. The three-dimensional representation proved most valuable, it was the first time that the complete network of the meridians could be studied as a system instead of piecemeal. A compendium written by Yang Ki-Cheou, the physician, and three meridian-statuettes dating from the Ming Dynasty (1368–1644) are the last relics of this prosperous period for acupuncture. The rulers of the following Dynasty (the Tsing, 1644–1911) had no trust in traditional medicine. This did not apply to the Chinese people and acupuncture and moxibustion continued to be practised, but they received no support in the field of research. The situation grew increasingly difficult in the days of cultural imperialism and during the Opium War (1840–42); finally, this school of medicine was prohibited by Decree. It had meanwhile become known in Europe and in Japan and was already being practised there.

Acupuncture in China subsequently received new support from the Communist Party; in 1928, at the time when the Red Army was created, Mao demanded full co-operation between traditional Oriental medicine and that of the West. During the Sino-Japanese War and on to the *Long March* to Jenan, acupuncture and moxibustion played an essential part in health care for the military. After the People's Republic had been proclaimed, both were able to win back their former place in the Research and Training Institutions of the country. Without the impetus given at that time, the giant stride into the future with the development of acupuncture anesthesia would never have been possible. Neither could one imagine the recent research in Laser Acupuncture being able to take place if this age-old inheritance of Chinese medicine had had to continue its existence as an outcast of modern science, relegated to practise in the doubtful shadows of a fair-ground tent.

The Techniques of Acupuncture and Moxibustion

This book, to be sure, is concerned solely with massage and acupressure for prevention and healing by the patient himself. Self-treatment obviously has its limits; there are cases when you have to consult a physician. You should always go to your family doctor in the first place. I am adding this brief digression for the attention of those who may be interested in acupuncture and pause to reflect on such elementary considerations as to whether it is painful, whether it is clean, whether it is really quite above-board . . .

I can do no more than describe the way acupuncture is operated, while giving no more information concerning the skill of the operator than would the theoretical description of an appendectomy concerning the skill of the surgeon performing it. If you should contemplate having recourse to acupuncture, always consult your doctor first and keep him informed as to the course and effects of the treatment. In the same way, tell the acupuncture specialist what treatment and what medicine have been prescribed to you to date, or what you may still be taking at the time of consulting him.

● In *acupuncture,* selected points of the anatomy, mainly situated on the meridians, are stimulated by means of needles made of gold, silver, or other metals. We use needles that are less than half a millimeter in diameter. The puncture varies in depths from a few millimeters to several centimeters according to the point of insertion; it is made at a carefully chosen angle to the body's surface, so that only an incorrect application by the operator or a sudden movement by the patient can produce discomfort, for instance by touching the wall of an artery, or may even injure an organ. There are several delicate points on which only experienced specialists are prepared to operate: for instance, to puncture the corner of the eye nearest to the nose, the needle must pass at a hair's breadth from the inner wall of the socket without touching the eyeball, a matter of fractions of a millimeter. That is why the training for acupuncture practicioners devotes so much time and care to the study of the human anatomy. The training includes a number of tests the student must carry out on his own person. These help him to acquire self-assurance and dexterity, as well as acquainting him by his own experience with the sensations produced by the manifold forms of acupuncture on which his patients will be reporting to him later on. It would be erroneous to imagine that the patient feels nothing, although any local discomfort is indeed almost invariably a sign of incorrect manipulation. Under correct professional treatment, what he will feel is the so-called *De Qi,* which means *the coming of energy.* Characteristic *De Qi* sensations are a sense of heat or cold, weight or pressure, irritation or electrification. There may be pain in some distant part of the body. Patients frequently report a sense of tension along the whole course of the meridian treated.

As regards local pain, I should specify that acupuncture at highly sensitive points, such as the finger tips or the soles of the feet, may cause slight discomfort to a sensitive patient. Persons who are nervous or anxious, or those being treated by acupuncture for the first time, are usually more likely to feel pain than is the habitué, who is well acquainted with acupuncture and has confidence in his operator.

After puncturing, the needles are usually left some fifteen to twenty minutes in position. The operator checks the position every few minutes and, as required by the treatment concerned, may move them from side to side, twist them between his fingers or set them vibrating. In emergency cases or during the intensive treatment of serious illnesses, needles may have to be left in the body for hours at a time and perhaps kept moving throughout this period until the required effect is produced.

The fine needles with their heads and points are not the only instruments used in acupuncture. In some cases it is

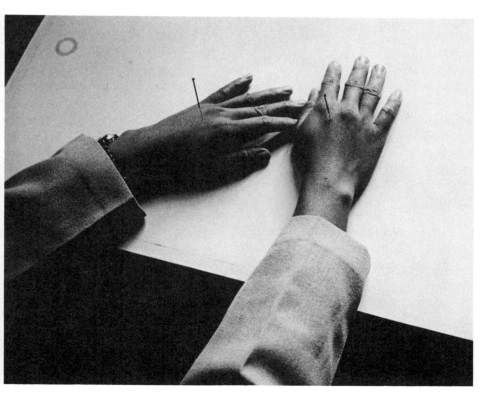

expedient to draw a small quantity of blood, usually by means of the lancets employed in conventional medicine to take blood from the finger tip. The technique called *Prunus blossom* is also widely used. A selected spot is tapped rhythmically with a small, long-handled cylindrical hammer having five to seven needles that have to be perfectly straight and applied vertically to avoid injuring the skin.

Cleanliness and sterilization of the needles have always been an essential and remain so more than ever nowadays when diseases transferred through the blood-stream, like hepatitis or AIDS, are so sadly prevalent. A hot-air oven, in which the needles are sterilized at 180° for a prescribed period of time, or other equivalent equipment, is part of the basic inventory of every acupuncture practice. Boiling, or disinfecting with alcohol, is not sufficient. On request, I naturally employ new needles. I also have regular patients who keep a set of needles of their own, which they take home with them in an alcohol solution and bring back when they return for treatment.

● The *Huangdi Nei Jing* recommends *Moxibustion* particularly for the treatment of disorders that arise from cold or humidity. In cases of fever, inflammation, high blood-pressure, this technique with its thermal effect is clearly unsuitable. In moxibustion, certain points of the anatomy, such as the navel, where acupuncture cannot be applied, are warmed with glowing tinder of dried and powdered wormwood leaves. In the past, wormwood Moxiballs used to be lit in direct contact with the skin; nowadays a slice of garlic or ginger-root is usually placed between them for insulation. The safest way to avoid any chance of burning the skin is "gentle moxibustion" with a moxi-stick. The operator lights the end of a stick of wormwood and, when it glows, holds it close to the skin and takes it away again at regular intervals. Thus the precise moment when the skin reddens as required can be easily observed. Heat therapy with wormwood (artemisia vulgaris) is used particularly in cases of fainting or debility, such as giddiness when the blood pressure is too low.

There is an old European tradition regarding the uses of wormwood. The soldiers of the Roman Legions are said to have put wormwood leaves in their sandals to ward off exhaustion on the long forced marches. It seems to have been specially connected with the feet. In German the plant is called *Beifuss;* it was used in a foot-bath for weary limbs. There are numerous wormwood prescriptions in traditional medicine, including cures for chronic diarrhea and for intestinal parasites. The main element in wormwood volatile oil is in point of fact cineol, which is a vermifuge. One wonders whether this property was known in the days when wormwood was one of the herbs put into a salad-dressing. The plant is a native of Europe as it is of Asia; independently of one another, both cultures had discovered its healing value at an early stage. Although this is only one example among many as concerns our common knowledge—not even a very good one, since conventional medicine has long replaced wormwood by chemical preparations, although it is still used in Western homeopathy,- it nevertheless gives me an opportunity to state my continued hope for growing cooperation between Western and Oriental medicine, highlighting further convergences in our traditions and above all seeking to progress together in research, to the end that the medical problems confronting us today may be solved.

THE PRACTICE OF
CHINESE MEDICINE

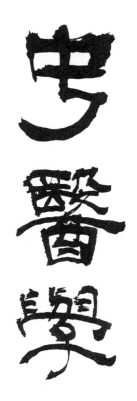

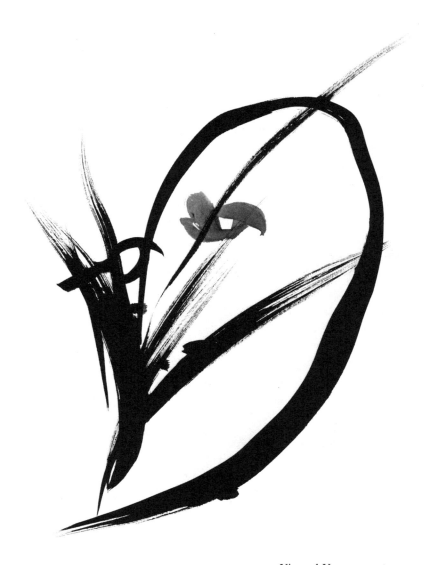

Yin and Yang are not antitheses that cannot meet. The slender bow symbolises Yin, but it broadens and merges into Yang.

The joy of a cancer patient on hearing from his doctor that after long years of arduous and painful treatment he was finally cured of his disease, was so great that he died of heart failure the same day in the course of a party he was giving his friends to celebrate the event. As seen by Western eyes, he should have left the organization of his party to someone else, instead of rushing round shopping and preparing everything himself. As I see it, he might have survived if he had taken his good news more calmly and had not been so entirely overcome with joy.

Yin and Yang, the two poles that determine all things in life, were thrown out of balance by this excessive joy. Uncontrolled emotions, whether positive or negative, are considered by Chinese medicine to be the primary germ of disease. As we see things, man is born perfect and invulnerable. It is by his own action that he turns his personal economy topsy-turvy, providing it with the wrong nourishment and gradually weakening his defence system as his life progresses. In a state of imbalance, he is more likely to fall ill in an extreme climate, or to be the victim of an accident, he is more prone to catch any infectious disease that may be about. Any loss of one's natural defences disturbs the energy flow, which we believe activates the human body and keeps it healthy. The channels by which energy flows through the body are called meridians. They are precisely located, they are the starting point of my treatment for a patient. If the energy flow is excessive, I can stem it. If it is insufficient, I can stimulate it. The diagnostic and therapeutic methods of Chinese medicine are based on the rules of the *Five Elements,* which influence nature and space, the human body and its organs, the humors and activities of man. *Fire* is the element of the heart and of joy; too much joy can exhaust the heart. *Wood* is the element of the liver and of anger. Fits of anger are harmful to the liver. The *Earth* rules the spleen and anxiety; the lungs and sorrow are subject to *Metal,* the kidneys and fear to *Water.* If we now think back and consider the case of the man who died of joy, it becomes clear why, in the opinion of an Oriental, he would have done well to practise more self-restraint.

The Rules of the Five Elements

In Ancient China, where daily life kept time to the work of the fields, awareness of the changing seasons led to the concept of the Five Elements with their varying energy flow. Spring, Summer, Late Summer, Autumn and Winter are the periods during which Wood, Fire, Earth, Metal, Water—these are called "Elements"—each in turn have their main energy output. Each element nourishes the next, just as each season produces the next. Each element not only nourishes but also has a restrictive influence on one of the others and thus the final energy balance remains steady.

These rules of genesis and decay were the old Chinese explanation for the interaction of repetition and change within time. One could be sure that the evening and the night would be followed by the new day and that the years would pass in accordance with the eternal laws.

Thus, men's minds were all the more troubled by any sudden change, some unexpected phenomenon—heat, rain, drought, wind or storm at an unusual time of year. A hot spring, for instance, meant that Fire, the summer element, had awakened too early and that was a bad sign. The natural order of things according to the *Rules of the Five Elements* was applied to various areas of human life, particularly in respect of health care. Each of the organs, heart, spleen, lungs, kidneys, liver, was seen as supplied by another, small intestine, stomach, large intestine, bladder, gall-bladder. The corresponding meridian-couples interact according to the rules of genesis and decay. That is why we never observe an affected organ by itself but only in its relationship to other organs or parts of the body that might have infected it, and which it might itself infect via the meridians and the five elemental energies. Precise

The Five Elements and Their Affinities in Man, in Nature and in Space

	WOOD	FIRE	EARTH	METAL	WATER
ORGANS:	liver	heart	spleen	lungs	kidneys
CAVITIES & TRACTS:	gall-bladder	small intestine	stomach	large intestine	bladder
SENSORY ORGANS:	eyes	tongue	lips	nose	ears
AWARENESS:	sight	taste	touch	smell	hearing
TISSUES:	ligaments, sinews	arteries	muscle	skin, body-hair	bones, head-hair
SECRETION:	tears	sweat	saliva	faeces	urine
TASTE	sour	bitter	sweet	sharp	salty
EMOTIONS	anger	joy	anxiety	sorrow	fear
EXPRESSION	shouting	laughing	singing	weeping	whimpering
TIME OF DAY:	morning	midday	afternoon	evening	night
LIFE CYCLE:	birth	growth	climacteric	decay	death
DIRECTION	East	South	Center	West	North
CLIMATE	windy	hot	damp	dry	cold
SEASON	spring	summer	late summer	autumn	winter
PLANET	Jupiter	Mars	Saturn	Venus	Mercury
COLOR	green	red	yellow	white	black
VEGETABLE FOOD:	corn	rice	maize	oats	beans
ANIMAL FOOD:	chicken	mutton	beef	horse	pork
METAL	tin	mercury	copper	iron	lead
SIGN	Dragon	Sun	Bird	Tiger	Moon-Tortoise

knowledge of these interrelationships is of great value in Chinese medicine. For instance, when we promote certain energies in the spring-time, we are taking preventive action in respect of summer complaints. Or, again, by treatment of the meridians, we are able to strengthen an organ that is threatened by a sick partner. The organs and their suppliers are connected two by two, each couple is ruled by one of the five elements,

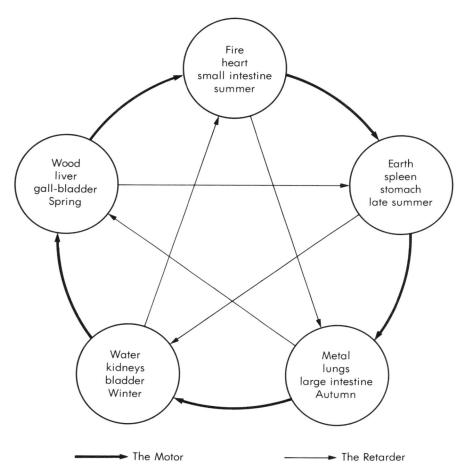

the energies of these determine the course of the seasons and the rules of promoting and restraining keep the circulation in a state of balance.

Yin and Yang

The concepts of Yin and Yang became familier to the West at a time when Chinese medicine had acquired some popularity there. I have noticed with regret that people have a very vague idea of what is meant by these two key terms. To be sure, the idea of two forces exerting a universal influence is extremely Chinese and perhaps not so easily acceptable elsewhere. On the other hand, I find that concepts and considerations in line with the Oriental school of thought are now being enunciated by Western thinkers with ever increasing clarity and this seems to me to be an endorsement of our own ideas. That man should preserve his inner balance, that violent emotions or unbalanced diet weaken our defenses, as now stated in recent publications,[*] have long been tenets of Chinese hygiene and are indeed based on the ancient Yin-Yang theory.

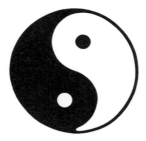

YIN (darkness) and YANG (light), the two forces penetrating all things, are not irreconcilable extremes; in every Yin there is also Yang, in every Yang there is Yin.

This doctrine, which obviously goes far deeper in its manifold strata, may be outlined as follows:

In the philosophy of Ancient China, the universe and all it contains are ruled by the two opposing forces of Yin and Yang. Basically, Yang means light and Yang, the opposite pole, means darkness. In time Yang came to denote the male, active element and Yin the female, passive one. The Earth was seen as Yin and Heaven as Yang. Thus Yang was above

---

[*] Cf. Mark P. Friedländer, Prof. Dr. Terry M. Phillips: *Für ein starkes Immunsystem,* Bern, 1987

and Yin was below. Finally, Yang and Yin became the generic terms for all that is diametrically different in nature, in outer space, in man.

For an Oriental, Man is an organic component of the universe. He is also an entity in himself, a microcosm where again all things are subject to Yin and Yang. His active life is Yang, his sleeping hours are Yin. The upper half of the body is Yang, the lower half is Yin. The arms are Yang, the legs are Yin. The digestive tract, an active producer of energy, is Yang. The heart, pericardium, lungs, liver, spleen, kidneys receive energy and are therefore Yin. Energy itself is Yang, the blood and the other body fluids are Yin. The inside of the body is Yin, its surface is Yang.

Yet, one should not be too categorical. These concepts are not cut and dried; Yin always contains some Yang and Yang always has a Yin component. The legs are Yin in relationship to the arms, but Yang in relationship to the rump. The liver is Yin, its surface is Yang. One and the same illness may be both Yang and Yin, progressive and then chronic. Yin and Yang are in fluid and not static equilibrium. Bearing in mind that the infinitely fine ramifications of the Yin-Yang network within the human body are reflected in just as many possible combinations in the mind and the spirit, in the environment and in the seasons, it becomes easily understandable that Chinese medicine should be so intensely concerned with prevention. An equilibrium as complicated as this is easier to preserve than to restore once it has been shaken. A balanced diet and harmonious inner life in an environment that is intact are the A and O for physical and mental health. It is not merely by chance that leading Oriental acupuncture specialists lay greater value on daily preventive massage than on the most sophisticated curative punctures.

A Chinese proverb says: "the good doctor treats diseases before they set in, the poor doctor afterwards." In the old days in China people might pay their physician as long as they were in good health; if they fell ill, he had failed in his task. I must say I find this somewhat exaggerated, although there is certainly something to say for the idea. I too find prevention most important, strengthening the body while it is in good condition. Chinese massage, practised daily, is an excellent defence against every-day ills and disorders. Acupressure too can frequently help ward off an illness by restoring the balance of the energy flow before worse things occur.

Diagnosis

Traditional Chinese medicine does not have recourse to X-Ray examinations or laboratory tests, endoscopy or biopsy or other precision techniques for diagnosis used in Western conventional medicine. The painstaking care and attention with which the Chinese doctor applies the media available to him for diagnosis must therefore be all the greater: these instruments are his own sensory organs.

Naturally, Western physicians—particularly general practicioners—depend largely on their observation of the patient. Both East and West, the relationship established between patient and physician has impact on the diagnosis and the choice of therapy. Has the patient sufficient confidence to discuss his problems frankly? Has the doctor taken the necessary time to observe the patient attentively and to talk with him? My Western colleagues and myself have the same initial duty, which is to begin by exhausting all the possibilities for diagnosis offered us in conversation with the patient without any outside intervention: looking, listening, smelling, asking questions, feeling and palpating.

This four-step diagnosis is offered the Chinese doctor in the form of a pre-established grid, enabling him to assess his findings according to the Yin and Yang principles and the laws of the Five Elements. His sensorial awareness is trained to use the grid. The acupuncture specialist must be able to see off-hand whether his patient's tongue tends to be "grayish," "brownish," or "yellowish." he must be able to judge the volume and tone of the voice. He should be able to note the "sweetish" or "sourish" smell of the patient's perspiration; and this is particularly difficult because most patients are careful to come to a consultation either smelling of nothing, or of bubble-bath or perfume. The patient fresh from a bath also complicates matters for the acupuncture practicioner because the body temperature and the state of the skin are influenced by the bath and these are both important items for the fourth step of the grid, where the doctor feels the pulse and palpates the patient's body.

By these four steps, seeing, listening and smelling, asking and feeling, Chinese medicine makes the diagnosis according to the Yin and Yang principles and the laws of the five elements. We do not seek for a disease to combat in the Western sense, we go further and seek the cause of the disease, that is to say the location and extent of the energy imbalance that is at the root of the disease. Thus the disease itself becomes a symptom. In acupuncture too, naturally, the doctor attacks the disease, relieves pain, reduces inflammation. However, he must assume that his therapy will be useless in the long run unless he can discover and remove the cause of the energy imbalance. So it is that acupuncture not only treats the disease but the patient's entire person. This means that the findings in diagnosis are not necessarily the same in the case of two patients who both complain of the same symptoms. The treatment also depends on the time of year and may vary on that account.

The clinical examination begins with detailed observation. The physician assesses the patient's constitution and his motility. He pays particular attention to the complexion, the color of the lips, the tongue, the eyes. In the teaching of the Five Elements these colorings provide information on the condition

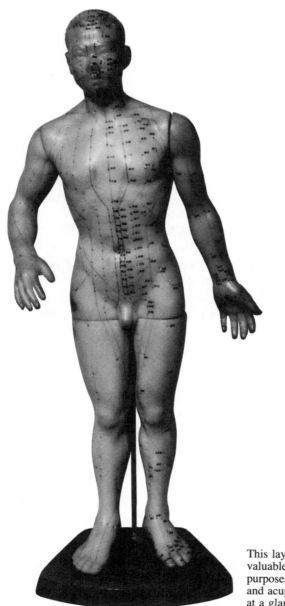

This lay-figure is most valuable for reference purposes. The meridians and acupoints can be seen at a glance.

of the body organs. They also tell him something more concerning the energy imbalance at stake.

The examination continues with listening and smelling. Is the patient's voice weak? Does he speak loud, fast, jerkily? What about his exhalation? Does his breath smell? Even though the symptoms may be hard to identify and interpret, they are just as important for diagnosis as the actual pains.

The third step is one of questioning. The physician asks the patient about his daily life, his habits, his past, his family. The patient should also speak of his illness and describe the way it has developed. It is important for him to locate any pains as precisely as possible. A headache, for instance, may be due to interruption of the energy flow along one of the meridians. There are connections between the stomach-meridian and pain in the forehead, between the gall-bladder meridian and pain in the temples, between the bladder meridian and pain in the back of the head and the nape of the neck, between the liver meridian and pain at the top of the head.

The clinical examination concludes with feeling the pulse and palpating the patient's body for painful or swollen places or points sensitive to pressure. The skin temperature is checked at the same time. In Chinese medicine a rise in temperature is considered as a combined symptom of a *vacuum* and *heat*. Cold sweat means a *vacuum* and *cold*. Hands and feet that are too hot denote a Yin-deficiency; if they are too cold it is a Yang-deficiency. The Chinese *pulse-diagnosis* demands much experience and an excellent sense of touch. The physician places his three fingers on three points of the pulse, one behind the other, on the patient's wrist. With three variations of pressure he then feels the surface pulse, the middle pulse and the deep pulse in all three places. He then compares his findings with those concerning the other wrist and lists them according to a number of characteristics. If the various pulses beat harmoniously together, the pulse as a whole is considered to be normal.

Western colleagues may perhaps find our diagnostic instrumentarium rather simple; actually it is extremely rich in information, as well as being highly exacting as regards the physician's sensorial awareness and affective comprehension, qualities which, to my mind and however sophisticated the existing technologies, are still the foundations of diagnosis.

The Eight Key-Symptoms

In the course of his four-step diagnosis the Chinese doctor has been approaching his patient gently and considerately. He has first observed him, listened to him and smelt him. Then he has asked him questions, ones that are easy to answer. Finally he has touched him, felt his pulse and palpated his body. To conclude, he must choose a therapy applicable not only to the disease but to the patient's entire person; to do this, he will classify the many findings of the clinical examination under the eight key-symptoms of Chinese medicine:

Depths	Surface
Cold	Heat
Emptiness	Fullness
Yin	Yang

These differentiations enable us to locate the energy disorder and determine the progression and severity of the ailment. One where the main symptoms are those of *emptiness* is likely to be of a chronic nature; emptiness indicates an energy deficiency. Symptoms of emptiness are for instance lack of appetite, night-sweat, a weak voice, lassitude. Symptoms of *Fullness* are phlegm (pituita), constipation, flatulence, dysenteric diarrhea and indicate an acute disorder. If the patient does not feel thirsty or prefers hot drinks, this is a symptom of *Cold*. Thirst for cold drinks, dry lips, red eyes, a general state of restlessness are symptoms of *Heat*. Pains in the limbs are *Surface* symptoms. Pains in the chest or abdomen point to a deep-lying energy perturbation.

Yin and Yang are the basic principles for the functioning of the whole organism. For this reason, any mal-function is Yin or Yang. *Depths, Cold* and *Emptiness* are the key-symptoms of a Yin disorder; *Surface, Heat* and *Fullness* are those of a Yang disorder.

The Chinese physician examines not only the disorder but also the patient according to the eight key-symptoms. Necessarily, this overall exploration leads him to select a therapy adapted to the individual. He may lay the main stress on diet or plant therapy. He may prescribe massage or acupressure. He may use acupuncture or the thermic techniques of moxibustion. In acupuncture he disposes of needles of many different shapes and made of many different materials. According to the patient's needs, he may apply additional needles at points not directly connected with the ailment but significant for the general condition. Delicate manipulation of the needles can stem or stimulate the energy flow as required.

However, all these many therapeutical possibilities in their various combinations, cannot detract from one other essential point: can we with our modest means assist the patient? Or is his illness one that needs treatment by conventional medicine? The Western school has highly powerful weapons to combat the most varied diseases. If this should be the case, we may be able to offer an analgesic, strengthening secondary treatment with no side-effects.

THE EIGHT WONDERS
OF CHINESE MASSAGE

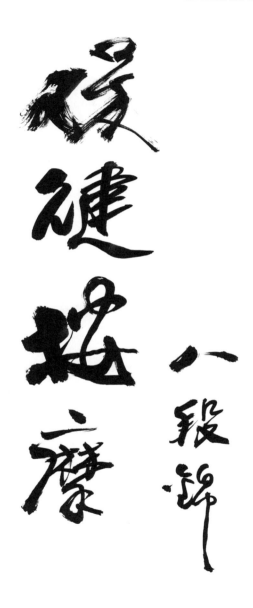

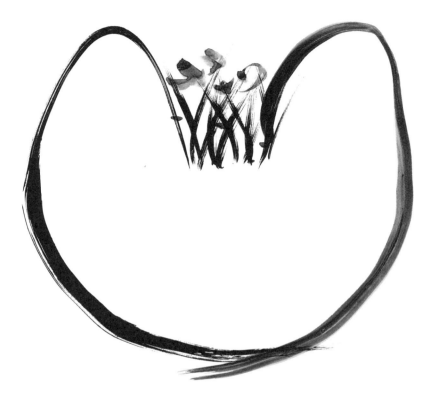

Massage is a soft and flowing thing, one that creates harmony—this is what the drawing has attempted to suggest.

Kan identifies the abysmal, water. In *I Ging,* the Book of Metamorphoses, we read under the sign Kan: "Water fulfils its aim by uninterrupted flowing. It fills all depths before flowing on." Let us retain this image of water, which I Ging quotes as an example for correct behaviour in certain situations, in our present discourse on massage. In the same way as energy should flow through the body, evenly and without interruption, our hands which influence the energy flow should glide over the skin: they should not skip over any hollow places, however shallow, but should apply the same pressure throughout. It is for you to decide how hard you will press. Even gentle stroking can work wonders, for the success of a massage depends on even pressure rather than intensity. Chinese massage is never forceful. It has nothing to do with any exhausting kneading of the muscles. Our bodies after all are more than a piece of dough to turn and pull into shape.

Chinese massage strengthens body and mind together. By stimulating the classical meridians, as well as other important areas outside their system, it vivifies the whole organism, having at one and the same time a preventive and a curative effect. It is more comprehensive than acupressure and acupuncture, which are aimed at the treatment of individual disorders. It is as easy as child's play, since it requires no knowledge of the exact position of the meridians or the acupoints. Furthermore, it can be done anywhere, without outside assistance. If you start applying Chinese massage regularly, you will soon find it an essential part of your daily physical hygiene. Concentrating on your body will be easier every time and, as you discover the *Eight Wonders* of the eight steps in massage, you will find out that there is also a Ninth, that of your own body, a small but perfect universe of its own.

"Is your nose stuffed up?" was the first question Dr. Kuan Hin asked me when I went to consult him. Of course my nose was not stuffed up; I had come for acupuncture, to cure my headaches. I wondered seriously whether I was doing the right thing.

In any case, I was not at all sure whether acupuncture would be of any use; I was simply trying it out, since I kept looking for some way to get rid of my headaches without medication. I had to travel to Paris on business pretty often and if Dr. Hin's needles turned out to be any good I could always come back for more. And now here I was and the man kept talking about my nose and insisting that it was stuffed up and I should massage it! And finally so I did and he showed me how and I was astonished at the results. I suddenly felt a great breath of air right through my head. My nose must have been stuffed up after all! When he asked "whether it was any better now," I was so overcome that I couldn't say a thing!

Dr. Hin showed me Inhoa-Massage and recommended that I should massage my head and face at any time during the day whenever I felt a headache coming. If I felt pain I should apply acupressure to the places where he then gave me acupuncture. This has not been necessary, for since I have learnt to use Inhoa-Massage daily the headaches have never returned in the same way again.

K.W., a travelling salesman,
Frankfurt-am-Main.

Preparation

You prepare for massage in three stages. First you get into the correct position. Then you concentrate. Finally you control your breathing by means of a few exercises.

Position: Make sure that you will not be disturbed during your massage. The best time to do it is either in the morning when you wake—particularly if you have difficulty in getting up!—or else in the evening before you go to bed; you will find it very easy to get to sleep after a massage. If you are in normal health, do it naked. It is a good opportunity to air your body properly. However, avoid being in a draught! As we say in Chinese, "keep out of the way of the wind and the flying arrow!" If you feel the cold, you can massage yourself under a blanket; the main thing is that the hands should be able to move freely over the body, flowing like water. Some massage is done seated, others lying down. It is up to you to choose the position you prefer. A complete massage will take you about half an hour.

Concentration: once you have taken up your position for massage, you must set your mind at rest. Forget your worries, forget your preoccupations. Forget your surroundings, hear nothing and see nothing. Your muscles are perfectly relaxed. You concentrate on two points of your body in turn. One is the special acupoint *Yintang,* just above the bridge of the nose in the center between the eyebrows. The other is the navel, which is surrounded with important acupoints; one is *Qihai,* the Sea of Energy (Ren-Mai meridian 6) and another is *Guanyuan,* the Pivot of Life (Ren-Mai meridian 4). The old masters said of these two points on the Ren-Mai meridian: "*Tan Tien* dwells in them." In traditional Chinese medicine, *Tan Tien* is the "Sea of Vitality," the "Gate of respiration," the "Root of the organs, the viscera and the meridians." When concentrating on *Yintang* and the navel, you should remember the following: if your blood pressure is low, concentrate mainly on *Yintang;* if it is high, concentrate mainly on the navel. Intense concentration on *Yintang* can cause the blood pressure to rise.

Breathing: for an Oriental, breathing permits an intake not only of oxygen but also of cosmic forces, of energy. Breathing is partly responsible for the success of a massage. There are two simple exercises to make your breathing calm and regular; it has to remain so throughout the massage. There are two kinds of abdominal breathing; one is natural, the other is the reverse movement much practised in the West. Use both forms and repeat each one three times, gradually increasing to twenty and then to thirty in the course of time.

Natural abdominal breathing: when you breathe *in,* the abdomen fills with air and is inflated, the chest rises slightly. When you expel the air, the abdomen contracts. If this exercise makes you feel ill, stop doing it. Rub the palms of your hands together, massage your face, take a few steps and drink a little warm water.

Reverse abdominal breathing: when you breathe in, you contract the abdomen and inflate the chest. When you expel the air, the chest subsides and the abdomen fills a little. While breathing in, press the tip of the tongue gently against the palate behind the canines; you breathe in through the nose. You then expel the air with your mouth open and the tongue returns to its place. For massage, take the breathing method that suits you best and seems easiest. Breathing exercises should not be overdone by persons whose respiratory organs or whose stomach is in poor condition, or during pregnancy. One's own feelings will be the best guide as to what is a good measure.

The First Wonder: The Dry Baths

The First Wonder consists in eight energetic massages, which we call dry baths. They come from a book written eight hundred years ago and called "The eight wonders of massage." The dry baths strengthen the whole organism. On the one hand they stimulate the circulation of the blood and ensure proper irrigation of the organs. On the other, they activate the energy flow and thus support the work of the digestive organs and the lymph system. This dual action on the blood (Yin) and on energy (Yang) will assist your body to maintain or restore its energy balance. The skin and the muscles are kept elastic and you feel fresh and at ease. Regular use of the *dry baths* will strengthen your defence system and you will be practising the supreme art of medicine, which is prevention.

The Hand-Bath: The hands are the initial or final points of six of the twelve regular meridians that are related to the organs. The three Yang-meridians of the hand run from the finger tips along the outer side of the arm to the head; the three Yin-meridians of the hand go from the chest along the inner side of the arm and the palm of the hand to the finger tips. The hand-bath stimulates the mobility of the finger joints and the sensitivity of the touch; it also prevents chapped hands. You massage incidentally and at the same time the meridian acupoints with their many therapeutical indications both on the palm of the hand with which you massage and on the back of the hand that you are massaging. Thus the Yin-meridians of one hand and the Yang-meridians of the other are always being massaged simultaneously.

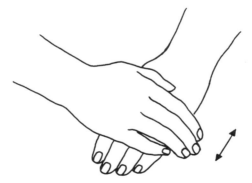

First rub the palms of the hands together until they are warm. Then grasp the wrist of one hand with the other hand and massage it over the back of the hand to the finger tips and back again. Repeat this massage sixteen times on each hand.

The Arm-Bath: The hand-meridians pass through the arm. The slightest infection can travel along them and be transmitted to the entire body. The Arm-Bath wards off inflammation by strengthening the vessels and keeping the wrist, elbow and shoulder supple. If you have any kind of infection in one arm, only massage the other. You can always treat a pain in the arm by massaging the corresponding part of your leg: the shoulder goes with the hip, the elbow with the knee and the wrist with the ankle.

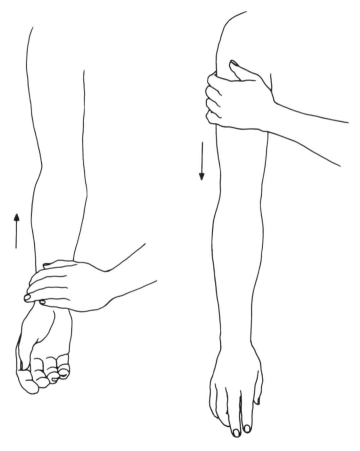

Put one hand on the inner side of the other wrist and slide it up the inner side of the arm to the shoulder, then over the shoulder and down to the wrist on the outer side. Massage each arm sixteen times.

Head-Bath: The head, which is the seat of the brain and the sensory organs, is doubtless the most sensitive part of the body. It is the junction of all the Yang-meridians and contains many acupoints that are outside the meridian system. The head should be massaged particularly gently to avoid reactoins such as giddiness or headache. You should stop massaging if you feel any kind of discomfort. The head-bath stimulates the circulation and input of oxygen. It strengthens your powers of concentration, your memory and your eyesight; it combats disorders of the speech-centers and paralysis phenomena.

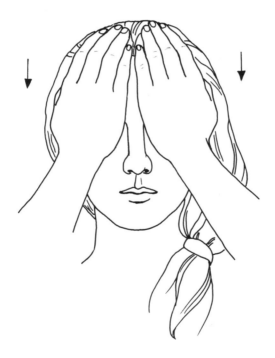

Put the palms of your hands vertically side by side on your forehead and move them down over your eyes, cheeks and mouth to the chin. Move on, on either side of the neck to the nape and up over the back of the head to the forehead. Repeat the movement sixteen times. If this is going to interfere

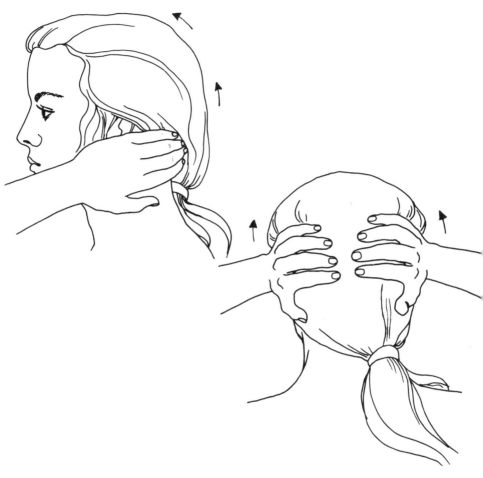

with your hair-do, move back from the chin to the forehead via the temples. If you also wear make-up, keep the whole massage for the morning when you are getting up, or the evening at bed-time. Finally, massage the temples with an upward movement towards the crown of the head until the fingers of your hands meet. Let your fingers interlock and move down over the center of the skull and the nape of the neck as far as you can. Repeat this massage sixteen times.

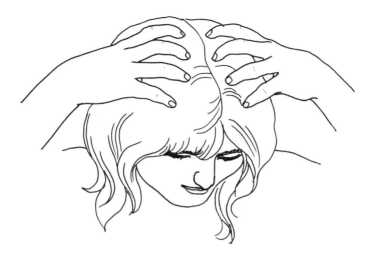

After massaging your face and the back of the head, massage your scalp, spreading your fingers and tapping gently with all the finger-tips at the same time. This should be repeated forty times, making sure that the four hundred delicate taps are evenly distributed over the whole of the scalp.

Nose-Bath: Speaking of the importance of this organ, the old Chinese masters used to say: "a stuffed-up nose is like a closed window." In point of fact, it is through the nose that we have access to the air and to the cosmic forces; it is an operative factor for our well being. Many of my patients have a stuffed-up nose, although they are unaware of the fact and are frequently astonished to find how much better they can breathe after nose-massage.

A stuffed-up nose is not only uncomfortable, it can lead to affections of the pharynx, or the lungs, or the bronchus. In our teaching, the lungs have a monitoring function in respect of the skin; skin damage may be connected with a stuffed-up nose. The Nose-Bath combats affections of the respiratory tract and also inflammation of the skin.

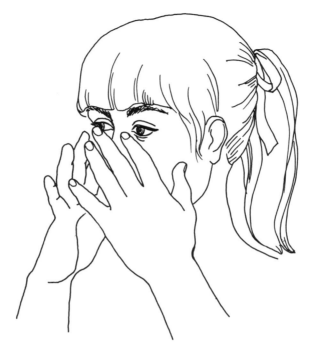

Put the tip of your first fingers or the back of your thumbs on either side of your nose and move up over the bridge to the forehead and back again forty times.

The nose with the many acupoints that surround it represents the whole human body. With a little imagination it can be compared to a human form, that of a child with the head between the eyebrows at the bridge of the nose, the body along the nose-bone, followed by the belly, and the thighs drawn up on either side at the nostrils.

Chest-Bath: The chest-bath strengthens heart and lungs physically; it can also relieve feelings of oppression and of fear.

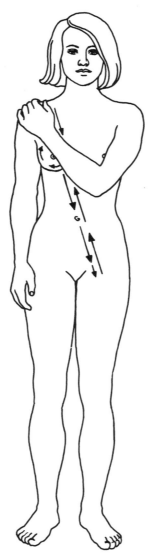

Place your left hand on your right shoulder, slide it down over the right breast, move round the nipple three times in a circle, then down in a diagonal to the left thigh. Return to the starting point. Massage both sides forty times each. Remember the image of water, that skips nothing and fills every hollow before flowing on.

Leg-Bath: Our legs are a place of transit for the three Yin-meridians and the three Yang-meridians of the foot. The leg-bath stimulates the circulation of the blood and activates the flow of energy in these meridians. It helps to keep ankles, knees and hips supple; it strengthens the leg muscles and prevents vascular fatigue effects (varicose veins, swollen feet). As usual, if there is an inflammation in one leg, only massage the other, or else the corresponding part of the arm.

Slide the palm of the hand from the groin to the ankle along the inner side of the leg and back again to the hip along the outer side. Massage each leg with an even pressure sixteen times.

Knee-Bath: Few joints have to stand as much wear and tear as our knees. There may be painful fatigue symptoms even when we are still quite young. There are few blood vessels in the knee, so it is particularly sensitive to the cold. It is frequently subject to inflammation. Massage keeps the knees supple and protects them from the cold. If you find massage painful, you can tap your knees gently with your fists instead.

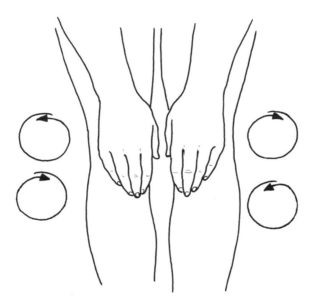

Rub your hands together to warm them; then massage both knees at the same time with a circular motion. Massage clockwise and anti-clockwise, sixteen times in each direction.

Eye-Bath: The eye-bath regulates the circulation of the blood and the energy flow, thus warding off numerous affections of the eyes. It keeps the eye muscles flexible and prevents premature crows' feet.

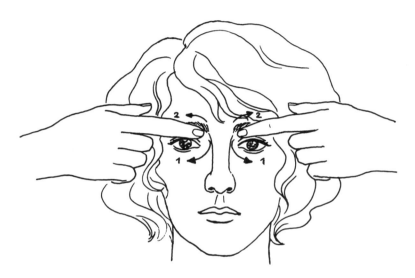

Massage both eyes simultaneously. Use the tip of the forefinger or the back of the thumb, as you prefer. Start at the corner of the eye nearest the nose, moving downwards and outwards, and go round the eye sixteen times before changing direction and doing another sixteen. This sequence is important, because, at the end of the massage, the skin over the bridge of the nose should be smooth and Yintang, the special point between the eyebrows, should be open. In conclusion, you move upwards from the inside corner of the eye and outwards over the eyelid.

There are two more massages, as a treatment for headache, to complete the Eye-Bath.

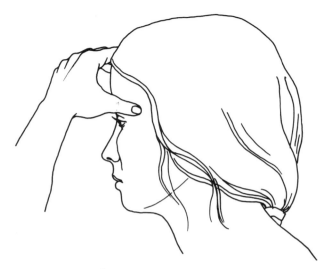

Massage your temples, circling over them with your thumbs, sixteen times in each direction.

Pluck at the point Yintang between the eyebrows with the thumb and forefinger of the right hand and then draw your thumb over your upper lip under your nose. While you are doing this, draw your left hand from the left temple over your forehead, top and back of your head, down the nape of the neck. Once you have completed this somewhat complicated exercise sixteen times, change hands and repeat it sixteen times more.

The Second Wonder: The Heavenly Drum

The ear, like the nose, represents the whole of man. Indeed, in auricular therapy every part of the organism is treated on the basis of the ear. Therefore there are a great many acupoints in the ear, over two hundred have been identified in the course of time. The *heavenly drum* massages these points, combats deafness and prevents otitis.

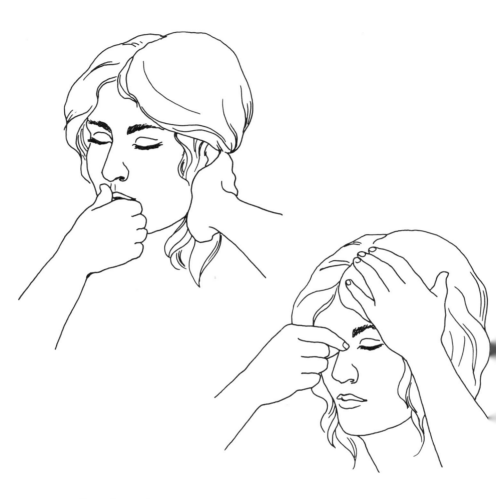

Put the palms of your hands over your ears and drum on the back of your head rhythmically with the forefinger, middle finger and ring-finger of both hands. Choose a fairly slow beat, such as your own walking pace. After the last beat, take your hands away quickly. Put your two forefingers into your ears, twist them about three times and pull them out with a jerk. Only do this exercise if your nails are trimmed short.

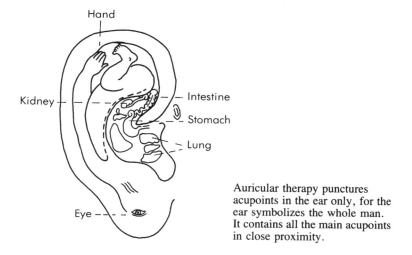

Hand

Kidney

Intestine

Stomach

Lung

Eye

Auricular therapy punctures
acupoints in the ear only, for the
ear symbolizes the whole man.
It contains all the main acupoints
in close proximity.

The Third Wonder: The Eye-Exercise

A Chinese physician can frequently assess the state of the
various organs from a person's outward appearance. The hair
reports on the kidneys, the skin on the lungs; the tongue
tells us about the heart and the eyes speak of the liver. If
there is any kind of eye trouble, the doctor will at once think
of an affection of the liver and will treat both together. The
Eye-exercise strengthens the eye muscles and the optic nerve.
We use it in various affections of the eye.

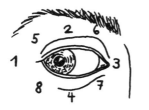 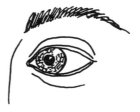

Whether you are seated or lying down, make sure that your back and your head are quite straight. Roll your eyes three times and then look right for a moment or two. After that, look straight ahead. Roll your eyes in the opposite direction and look left. Repeat the exercise and look upwards, downwards and finally in each diagonal direction.

The Fourth Wonder: Exercise for the Teeth

In Chinese teaching, the teeth are in direct relationship not only to the bones and tissues but also to certain organs. This exercise strengthens the jaws and the teeth and is good for the digestive system. Furthermore, it entails a delicate, vitalizing tapping at the brain and helps to clear your head.

You must keep your mouth shut and completely relaxed. Gnash your teeth very slowly forty times.

The Fifth Wonder: Rinsing the Mouth

The value of saliva as a disinfectant and an antidote is known instinctively to every child, who will always suck a damaged finger, whether at home in the valley of the Nile, on the Yangtzekiang, in New England or a village in Switzerland. Knowledge of the antiseptic properties of spittle has been part of human medicine from time immemorial. In China spittle is synonymous to life: the character meaning *Life* is made up of two components, *fluid* and *tongue*.

Rinsing the mouth facilitates digestion and wards off infection of the buccal cavity. Practiced together with the exercise for the teeth, it combats caries and strengthens the muscles of the jaws. You do it like this:

Keep your mouth shut with the upper and lower teeth touching. Move your tongue about, as though you were rinsing your mouth with water. Swallow the saliva that this produces in three parts. Repeat the movement forty times. When you swallow, imagine that the salvia is a solid, sliding down into the stomach.

Lao-Tze says that what is softest on earth overcomes what is hardest. Our massage is a soft, gentle art, seeking harmony, working to set flowing what is obstructed, to restore balance to what is out of gear. The more serious an affection, the easier it will be to heal it by this gentle means.

The Sixth Wonder: Renal Massage

The purpose of renal massage is to protect the kidneys, and more specifically the *renal eyes,* situated on the Dai Mai, a special meridian that encircles the waist like a belt at kidney level. These *eyes* have to be protected from cold, which they abhor; they need warmth and are highly sensitive to fluctuations in temperature. Renal massage harmonizes the circulation of the blood and the flow of energy and it keeps the temperature steady. Thus it relieves backache and has a preventive action as regards rheumatism. Its harmonizing action is also beneficial to the sexual organs. Renal massage may restore menstruation regularity and relieve or even entirely cure menstruation pains. It is a useful adjuvant in treatment for impotence.

During pregnancy, you should be very careful in using renal massage and particularly as regards the idea of creating warmth. If there is any kind of inflammation of the kidneys, refrain from using it at all; warmth could make the trouble worse.

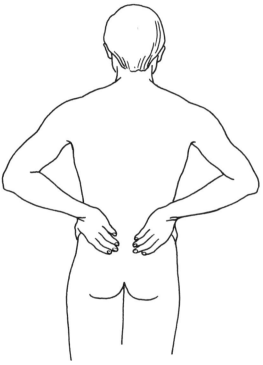

Rub the palms of your hands together until they are really warm and press them on your kidneys, imagining to yourself a pleasant stream of warmth flowing from your hands to your back and into the "renal eyes." Concentrate on this energy exchange up to two minutes. Then slide your hands down to the coccyx and back up the spine as far as you can go. Repeat this massage forty times.

The Seventh Wonder: Abdominal Massage

Abdominal Massage stimulates five meridians simultaneously, those of the stomach, the spleen, the kidneys, the liver and the special meridian, Ren-Mai. The stomach-and spleen-meridians fortify the digestive tract and stimulate intestinal activity; they have preventive action in respect of various affections such as gastric ulcers, constipation or diarrhea, spasms. Ren-Mai governs all the Yin-Meridians and runs down the body through the center of the trunk. It controls the body-fluids, making sure that not a drop should leave the system unnecessarily. When you stimulate it, you are fortifying the immunity-system and the sexual organs. When you stimulate the kidney-and liver-meridians, you are regulating bladder activity and preventing abdominal disorders.

It stimulates a meridian, simply to pass your hand over it; however simple and inadequate abdominal massage may appear to an outsider, you will find its action manifold and most beneficial.

In view of the differences in our anatomy and the specificity of our sexual requirements, men use one comprehensive circular motion for this massage while women massage the area of the stomach and that of the belly separately, out of consideration for their sensitive internal sexual system.

A note of warning! Abdominal massage may prevent a gastric ulcer, but if you have one already you must avoid it entirely! In the same way it must be avoided in cases of appendicitis or peritonitis and of all types of cancer in the abdominal area. Do not use it either, if you have been fasting for a long period, or if on the other hand you have just had a heavy meal. Both extremes should be avoided in any case.

Abdominal Massage for women: *Put your right hand under your left breast and massage the stomach area in a circular motion, clockwise, with its lowest point just above the navel. Repeat forty times. Then put your left hand just below the navel and massage the abdomen in a circular motion, anti-clockwise, forty times. Massage gently, almost without pressure. This is particularly important in pregnancy and for elderly women.*

Abdominal Massage for men: *Put your right hand under your left breast and massage the entire abdominal area, clockwise, forty times, in one broad circular motion. Then put your left hand under your right breast and repeat the massage forty times anti-clockwise.*

If you do this massage lying down, let the hand that is not busy lie relaxed. If you are seated or standing, put your hand to your waist on the same side of the body, with the thumb in front and the fingers in the small of the back. This position stretches the upper part of the trunk and gives you a wider expanse to massage.

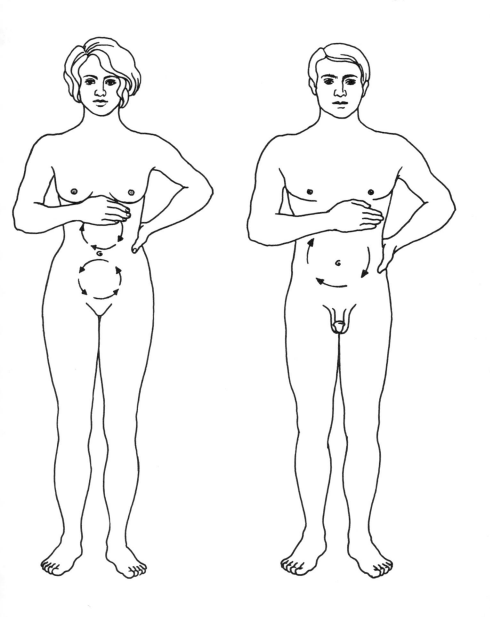

The Eighth Wonder: The Massage of the Gushing Spring

Yongquan—the gushing spring—is the name given to the first acupoint on the kidney-meridian, running from the sole of the foot along the inner side of the leg and over the belly to end under the shoulder-blade. The *gushing spring* deserves its name; it lies in the hollow just beyond the center of the sole towards its outer edge, and it repeatedly proves itself a friend in need, to which the acupuncture operator has recourse in cases of shock, unconsciousness and epileptic fits.

The feet are further away from the heart than any other part of the body. Circulatory troubles are frequent. In Chinese massage we use the gushing spring to activate the circulation of the blood and to prevent swollen feet, vascular disorders, cramp in the calves, and other unpleasant sequellae of irrigation deficiency.

Like all the other acupoints that lie lower than the knee or beyond the elbow, the gushing spring has preventive and therapeutic powers that extend far beyond the local area. It prevents nephitis, it strengthens the liver and, in conformity with the *laws of the elements,* it likewise strengthens the eyes. It relieves abdominal pains, combats coughing, hoarseness and sore throat, and it has a sedative effect in case of palpitations or distress.

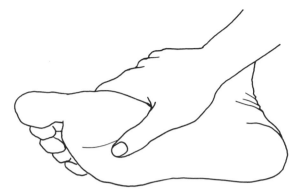

Place your right foot on your left knee. Grasp your foot with your right hand and massage the gushing spring with your thumb. Massage with a circular motion forty times, clockwise and anti-clockwise in turn. Then repeat the massage with your left thumb on your left foot.

ACUPRESSURE: HEALING WITH THE HANDS

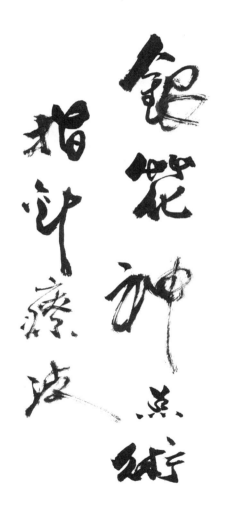

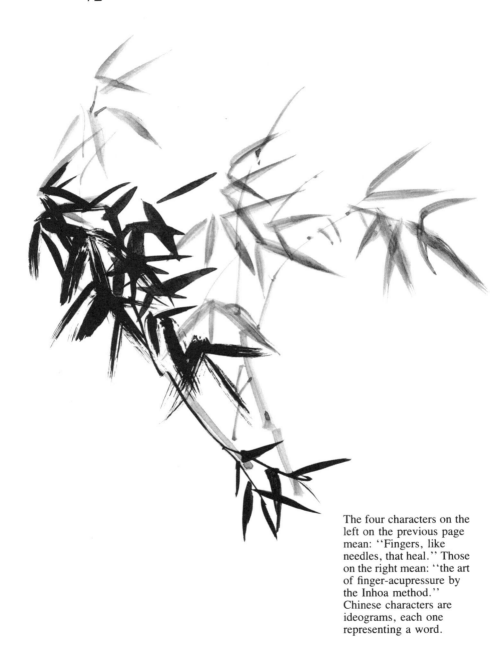

The four characters on the left on the previous page mean: ''Fingers, like needles, that heal.'' Those on the right mean: ''the art of finger-acupressure by the Inhoa method.'' Chinese characters are ideograms, each one representing a word.

Perhaps you have been having a look at the illustrated section of this book and wondering how it is that the same acupoints keep re-appearing for the treatment of many different diseases and complaints. You may have wondered why one and the same point is sometimes shown as the central point and sometimes as an ancillary one. This is not however a sign of confusion, but rather one of intentional therapeutic concatenation, whereby we are attempting to combine the action of the individual meridians and acupoints to the best possible advantage. Since the meridians and the organs obey the laws of the Five Elements and can heal or harm one another mutually, a disease can only be attacked at the root if its treatment likewise prevents possible infection elsewhere in the body. Thus, each point has a different, specifically curative or preventive function. And as most of the acupoints in Chinese medicine have more than one field of action in therapy, their functions may be re-formulated from case to case. Like the figures on a Chessboard, they find themselves faced with new tasks of defence or attack according to situations in continual change.

Chinese children are taught massage and acupressure while they are still very young. The sooner they get to know their bodies and the energy that flows through them, the sooner they will be able to interpret even insignificant alarm signals of energy imbalance and the sooner too they will be able to deal with minor every-day complaints, indigestion, a headache, or a cold in the nose. Together with dietetics and personal hygiene, daily self-applied massage and the rudiments of acupressure are the foundations of Chinese preventive medicine.

Knowledge of the interior relationships, the manifold direct and indirect interaction between the meridians and the organs of the body, is reserved for specialists in China. For the Oriental, and certainly for the Western uninitiated, the criteria, whereby the acupuncture specialist selects and elaborates a set of points for puncture, usually remain a mystery. The specialist himself remains a student all his life, continually analysing his successes and his failures, constantly discovering new combinations for acupuncture. To be sure, we have text-books with the detailed description of therapy using hundreds of acupoints. Yet, even if we may have treated an illness successfully with a particular set of points, how are we to know whether there might not be a yet more successful variant that has not yet been discovered? Again, I am thinking of a game of Chess. The champion may well have more than a thousand games stored in his memory and yet his final, winning move may be one that has never been played before.

My recommendations for acupressure in respect of individual complaints should be seen in this light. They are based on the doctrine of a medical School that is over a thousand years old, on the medical knowledge of my ancestors that was handed down to me, and on my own experience after practising for a number of decades. However, the therapy I can suggest is not the last word. Above all, acupressure cannot—nor does it seek to—compete with Western medicine and cannot be employed as a substitute for it.

The Acupuncteur treats his patients individually on the basis of the indications given him by the Chinese diagnostic matrix, selecting the main acupoints for therapy and adding to them or varying them according to individual requirements. He does not treat disease as an isolated symptom but as part of a whole, the energy system of an individual person that is temporarily off balance.

You may be wondering whether there is any point in a book on Acupressure, which obviously cannot take up the individual problems and requirements of its readers. The recommendations in it provide precisely the type of fundamental outline I have just been talking about. In some cases they may provide an adequate cure; in others they will need the support of more far-reaching forms of therapy. I do not mean necessarily adding other acupoints; it might be a change in eating habits, in attitudes in one's occupation, multiple factors in one's way of life that could have led to the disease in question. There are forms of therapy you have to prescribe for yourself; if you take the trouble of scrutinizing your body and your mind, you may be able to put your finger on the sore spot before an illness actually breaks out.

Acupuncture and Acupressure are based on the same teaching and experience, the points treated are the same in both methods. Acunpuncture is more effective, the therapy is more far-reaching; I also endeavour to keep my own energy flow wide open when treating a patient; that is why I cannot look after an unlimited number of people on the same day. Acupressure has other advantages; the patient can apply it himself, at any time and in any place, almost as often as he likes. That is why I show many of my patients how to use it, even if it is only as an adjuvant.

"I was in Switzerland, at Bad Schinzach, to convalesce after a serious knee-injury due to a motoring accident. The knee had been operated successfully, but I was not to put my weight on it for several weeks; I was indeed incapable of walking, except with crutches; the muscles were in very poor condition.

I heard of Dr. Hin, because he was at the same hospital at that time and was said to be working wonders; I was sceptical and in any case I saw no reason why he should treat me, since my recovery would be only a matter of time.

Nevertheless, one day I happened to get into conversation with Dr. Hin and I spontaneously told him my story. He at once said: "I will give you treatment for your knee; you will then be able to walk as you did before the accident." I agreed somewhat unwillingly, not at all sure what I was in for. After the Doctor had placed his needles at various points of my anatomy, I felt a fortifying warmth, surging and flowing in my injured leg. I had imagined that the treatment would be painful and unpleasant, whereas it was a unique experience, an awareness of power such as I had never dreamt of before.

After a few minutes, Dr. Hin extracted his needles and told me to start walking. It was an unnecessary injunction, for I could feel that I could now put the crutches away for good. I could walk normally without any kind of discomfort and I went straight out and through the hospital grounds to the newspaper-stand, where I ran into the surgeon-in-charge, who could not believe his eyes and finally told me to go back to bed for fear of complications with my insurance policy.''

H.G., an actress,

Bern

The Meridians

Vitality is made up of three types of energy:
genetic energy which dates from our conception and is equipped with the physical, mental and spiritual capabilities of our ancestors;
nutrient energy which is produced by the functioning of our digestive system;
cosmic energy which we receive from the atmosphere as we breathe.

This tripartite energy flows through a system of meridians and their ramifications in a steady twenty-four hour cycle, pervading every part of the body and ensuring the proper functioning of the organism.

The meridians of Chinese medicine are classified in two groups. One contains the twelve regular meridians of "hand" and "foot"; these cover an identical network on the right-hand and left-hand side of the body and are Yin or Yang in character according to that of the organs with which they are connected and after which they are named. The second group contains eight special meridians, not connected with any particular organ. Two of these special meridians are particularly important for therapeutic routine, because they monitor the twelve regular meridians and are studded with a large number of important acupoints. Together with the twelve regular meridians, these two form *the fourteen classical meridians of Chinese medicine.*

The Twelve Regular Meridians

In antiquity the Chinese learnt by experience that pressure on certain points of the body's surface had a curative effect in the treatment of certain illnesses. They soon saw that certain combinations of such points could heal disorders of specific organs. The relationships between the body functions and these points (*Xue,* "a point") led to a system on which the complex system of the meridians was built up step by step.

Twelve organs gave their names to the regular meridians; six of them are Yin and are "full"; they are guardians and distributors of energy. The other six are Yang; they are "hollow" and produce energy. In the list below, we have called the first set *organs* and the second cavities (or hollow organs):

Organs (Yin)	Hollow organs (Yang)
Lungs	Large intestine
Heart	Small intestine
Pericardium	Tripartite Warmer
Spleen	Stomach
Kidneys	Bladder
Liver	Gall-bladder

As already stated, the theory of the meridians is not founded on the organs themselves but on their function. The fact that our list includes an area in the abdominal cavity called "the tripartite warmer" is typical of the differences that may exist between the Western and the Oriental concept of the body functions. A brief survey of these functions as seen in Chinese medicine may help you to a clearer understanding of the meridians and their properties.

The lungs are connected with the outside air by the trachea and the nose. They have action on the skin and the body-hair. They govern energy, breathing and the discharge of water. Their characteristic property is one of collapse. They control all the respiratory organs and regulate the body fluids and the circulation of the blood. The relevant complaints are subject to the lungs.

The large intestine transports solid waste and processes it into faeces which are finally discharged via the anus.

The heart houses the spirit, the blood and the meridians. Its condition is shown by that of the tongue. It is related to the cortex and the cardiovascular system of Western medicine. Complaints of these are subject to the heart. The pericardium is the protective outer wall of the heart. Heart disease is frequently due to the pericardium being attacked by feverish disorders and unable to function properly.

The small intestine redigests for the second time whatever it receives from the stomach. It separates nutritive substances from waste, assimilates them and nourishes the whole body via the spleen, which transfers them to heart and lungs. The waste is sent on to the large intestine for discharge. Its overall function is the sorting-out of good and bad.

The pericardium is the heart's rempart. To reach the heart, any attack has to pass it and it has to stand in for the heart to receive whatever disease it may be. At the same time, the pericardium is a gate, the entry and exit of whatever concerns the mind, which is centered in the heart. Spiritual disorders and their symptoms concern not only the heart but also the pericardium.

The tripartite warmer is the name given to an area covering three levels of the abdominal cavity; it is the transformer-station for the body, where the organic activities are turned into energy. The tripartite warmer must work properly if the organs are to function and carry out their tasks in the transport and distribution of energy, blood, fluids, the assimilation of nourishment, the discharge of waste and so on.

The spleen controls nourishment, transports the body fluids and combats humidity. The causes of disorders of the digestive system and the circulation are connected with the spleen. The main properties of the spleen are to shun humidity and to seek dryness.

The stomach receives, distributes and digests food. Whereas the spleen monitors transport, the stomach processes food and is the central organizer of its distribution. Unlike the spleen, the stomach seeks humidity and shuns dryness wherever possible.

The kidneys are the store for essences and energy. They monitor reproduction, secretions and the urinary system. They are the "matrix of bone-marrow," they control the bones and are linked with the brain. Their connection with the outside world is via the ears. Their condition may be assessed by that of the hair. Symptoms of disease in all these parts are related to the kidneys.

The bladder is the collector and discharge-point for urine. It transforms energy and draws off excess water. Since the bladder is linked to the kidneys, their respective diseases interact.

The liver is the store-room for the blood. It monitors the articular ligaments and controls the circulation of energy. Its state is shown in the eyes. According to Chinese doctrine, the liver-system likewise embraces that of the nerves and certain secretions. The causes of disease in these parts are connected with the liver. Eye trouble too often goes hand in hand with a mal-function of the liver.

The gall-bladder is subject to the liver and various disorders are common to both. It is the part of the digestive tract where the bile is stored and distributed. A simultaneous excess of heat and humidity in the body can cause such imbalance in the gall-bladder that there will be an outbreak of jaundice.

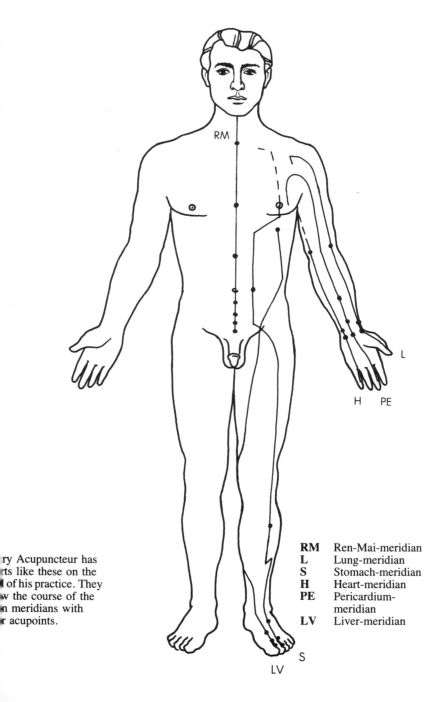

RM

L

H   PE

S

LV

Every Acupuncteur has charts like these on the wall of his practice. They show the course of the main meridians with their acupoints.

RM	Ren-Mai-meridian
L	Lung-meridian
S	Stomach-meridian
H	Heart-meridian
PE	Pericardium-meridian
LV	Liver-meridian

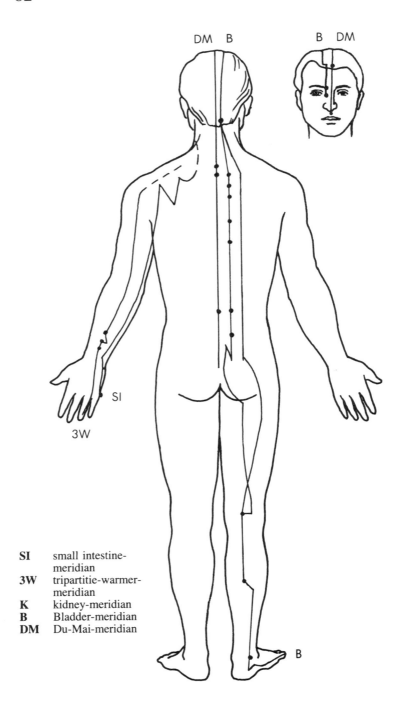

SI small intestine-
meridian
3W tripartitie-warmer-
meridian
K kidney-meridian
B Bladder-meridian
DM Du-Mai-meridian

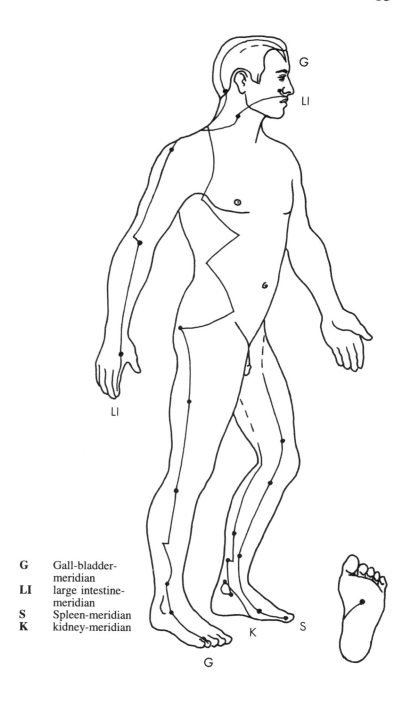

G   Gall-bladder-
          meridian
LI   large intestine-
          meridian
S   Spleen-meridian
K   kidney-meridian

The main functions of the twelve organs and corresponding cavities and channels as described show that the meridians do not simply begin in particular organs and end somewhere on the surface of the body, but are linked with one another in a network of mutual impact and interdependency. The course of a meridian does not necessarily run closer to the organ or cavity that has given it its name than to any other, at any rate not in the surface-area where its stimulation takes place. We may understand the meridians as being the functional images of organs and cavities, that pursue a given course on the body surface and therefore—unlike the deep-lying parts— are subject to influence by means of acupuncture, moxibustion, acupressure and massage.

The twelve meridians reach the furthest points of the four extremities. For some of them, the finger-tips or the toes are their goal, for others their source. The six Yin-meridians of the organs go along the inner side of the arms and legs, the six Yang-meridians of the cavities follow the outer side of the limbs. Every Yin-meridian is connected with a Yang-meridian by a ramification, a disorder of either may affect the other.

Organs	Cavities
The three Yin-meridians of the hand go from the chest to the hand along the inner side of the arm.	*The three Yang-meridians of the hand go from the hand to the head along the outer side of the arm.*

Lung ⟵——————————⟶ large intestine
Heart ⟵——————————⟶ small intestine
Pericardium ⟵——————————⟶ tripartite warmer

The three Yin-meridians of the foot go from the foot to the head along the inner side of the leg.	*The three Yang-meridians of the foot go from the head to the foot thru the rump and the outer side of the leg.*

Spleen ⟷ stomach
Kidneys ⟷ bladder
Liver ⟷ gall-bladder

The Yin- and Yang-meridians are coupled in pairs by means of ramifications. To ensure balanced circulation of energy, additional links are necessary between the meridians of the hand and those of the foot. Every Yin-meridian of the hand has its Yang partner and is also linked with a Yin-meridian of the foot. The same applies in reverse to every Yang-meridian and thus the circulation finally follows the following channels:

1. Lung-meridian of the hand—Taiyin
2. Large intestine-meridian of the hand—Yangming
3. Stomach-meridian of the foot—Yangming
4. Spleen-meridian of the foot—Taiyin
5. Heart-meridian of the hand—Shaoyin
6. Small intestine-meridian of the hand—Taiyang
7. Bladder-meridian of the foot—Taiyang
8. Kidney-meridian of the foot—Shaoyin
9. Pericardium-meridian of the hand—Jueyin
10. Tripartitie-Warmer-Meridan of the hand—Shaoyang
11. Gall-bladder-meridian of the foot—Shaoyang
12. Liver-meridian of the foot—Jueyin

The Course of the Twelve Regular Meridians and Their Disorders

If a meridian does not fulfil its physiological task, which is the circulation of energy and blood, its partner organ or cavity may be damaged and there may also be symptoms of disease along its path. For instance, functional disorder of the large intestine-meridian may lead to trouble in the large intestine, but it may also give you toothache, because the large intestine-meridian passes through the gums of the lower jaw.

Functional disorders of the meridians may have external

or internal causes, so we must discuss endogenous and exogenous illnesses.

Endogenous illnesses are due to dis-harmony of the emotions: anger, joy, anxiety, sorrow, fear are out of balance. Endogenous complaints first affect the organs or cavities and subsequently the meridians concerned; they are harder to treat than exogenous disorders.

Exogenous illnesses arise from climatic factors, too much heat or wind, humidity, aridity or cold. In their early stages, exogenous complaints affect the meridians; they have to be treated quickly, before they attack the organs and cavities concerned. The linkage and the symptoms of disease of the indivdiual meridians may be seen from their course.

The Lung-Meridian of the Hand—Taiyin

The lung-meridian starts in the abdominal cavity on the middle level of the tripartite warmer. it goes down to the large intestine, then up to the stomach and leaves the abdomen via the diaphragm. It divides to pass through both lungs, rises in the neighborhood of the trachea and reaches the surface for the first time at the outward end of the collar-bone, where we find the first acupoint of the lung-meridian. It goes down the inner side of the arm, passes the wrist, where it is the foremost of the three Yin meridians of the hand, and goes along the ball of the thumb to the tip, where it ends. Between the shoulder and the tip of the thumb, there are eleven acupoints having direct impact on the lung-meridian. A ramification from the wrist links it to the forefinger and thereby to the large intestine-meridian, which is its Yang partner.

Symptoms of disorders: feelings of oppression, coughing, breathlessness, hemoptysis, sore throat, cold in the head, pain in the shoulder-blades, or feeling cold there, pains in the meridian area.

The Large Intestine-Meridian of the Hand—Yangming

The large intestine-meridian runs from the tip of the forefinger to the metacarpus and up the outer side of the arm to the shoulder; it is the foremost of the Yang-meridians of the hand. From the shoulder it is diverted to the seventh vertebra, where it meets all the other Yang meridians, then it enters the hollow over the collar-bone and goes down via the lungs to the large intestine, where it is no longer accessible from outside. A ramification with important acupoints rises from the collar-bone hollow to the throat and the cheek, crossing the central vertical body-line between the upper lip and the nose and ending at the side of the nose, where it joins the stomach-meridian. The large intestine-meridian has twenty acupoints between the forefinger and the nose.

Symptoms of disorders: abdominal pains, diarrhea, constipation, sore throat, toothache, nose-bleeding, pains in the meridian area.

The Stomach-Meridian of the Foot—Yangming

The first acupoint of the stomach-meridian lies just below the eye. Its path runs from there to the gums of the upper jaw, the corner of the mouth and the chin, to the mandibular joint. A ramification runs straight from the jaw to the collar-bone, where it goes down inside the body to the stomach, the main tract of the meridian passes the chest at the nipple, enters the abdominal area, approaches the central body-line and reaches the thigh via the abdomen. At this point a ramification takes over, after starting from the stomach and going down the front of the leg and the instep to the second toe. Another ramification branches off below the knee and leads to the middle toe. A third ramification goes from the instep to the big toe and serves as a link to the spleen-meridian.

The stomach-meridian is the only Yang-meridian from the foot over the front of the body. It has forty-five acupoints.

Symptoms of disorder: Flatulence, stomach pains, edema, vomiting, swellings, pains in the throat, nose-bleeding, feverishness, mania, pains in the meridian area.

The Spleen-Meridian of the Foot—Taiyin

The spleen-meridian starts at the big toe and runs the whole length of the foot, following the color-line between the sole and the upper part, to the ankle, it then rises along the shinbone and up the inner side of the thigh into the abdomen, whence it reaches the spleen, which gives it its name. From the spleen it continues upwards to the chest, passes to one side of the nipple to the armpit, where it again takes a sideways turn, ending in the sixth inter-costal space below the armpit, where its last acupoint is located. It has a ramification going up the esophagus and ending under the tongue. A second ramification passes over the stomach and through the diaphragm to the heart, linking the spleen-meridian with the heart-meridian.

The spleen-meridian has twenty-one acupoints.

Symptoms of disorders: painful stiffness of the tongue, stomach pains, flatulence, vomiting, jaundice, general debility, pains in the meridian area.

The Heart-Meridian of the Hand—Shaoyin

The heart-meridian begins in the heart, crosses the lung and reaches its first acupoint on the body surface in the center of the armpit. Among the three Yin-meridians of the hand, it is the one furthest from the front; it goes down the inner side of the arm to the wrist and thence in a straight line over the palm of the hand to the tip of the little finger, where it joins its Yang partner, the small intestine-meridian. There is a ramification from the heart through the diaphragm to the small intestine and another that leads to the head and ends at the eye. The heart-meridian can be stimulated at nine acupoints.

Symptoms of disorders: dryness of the throat, pains in the region of the heart, hot hands, pains in the meridian area.

The Small Intestine-Meridian of the Hand—Taiyang

The small intestine-meridian goes from the little finger over the back of the hand to the wrist-bone. Among the three Yang-meridians of the hand it is the one furthest from the front; it goes up to the elbow and along the outer side of the arm to the shoulder. Passing over the shoulder-blade it reaches the seventh vertebra, where it meets the other Yang-meridians. Crossing the shoulder, it reaches the hollow over the collar-bone and goes straight from there to the heart. Finally it runs up the esophagus, then down to the stomach and the spleen, where it belongs. There is a ramification running from the collar-bone sideways across the neck to the cheek and another that branches off from the cheek and passes under the eyeball through to the inner corner of the eye, where it joins the bladder-meridian.

The small intestine-meridian has nineteen acupoints.

Symptoms of disorders: Belly pains, deafness, jaundice, cheek tumors, throat pains, pains in the meridian area.

The Bladder-Meridian of the Foot—Taiyang

The bladder-meridian starts at the inner corner of the eye and runs up over the forehead to the crown of the head. A ramification goes from the top of the head to the temples and the meridian itself briefly enters the brain and goes down the back of the head to the neck. It runs parallel to the spine as far as the small of the back where it first enters the kidneys and then reaches the bladder. One branch goes from the sacrum to the hollow of the knee via the buttocks and the back of the thigh. There it is joined by a further ramification which had left the main meridian at the nape of the neck and reached the buttocks before it at a somewhat greater distance from the spine. This last ramification completes the path of the bladder-meridian, going down the calf behind the outer ankle-bone to the instep and along the outer edge of the foot to the little toe. There it links with the kidney-meridian.

We have access to the bladder-meridian at sixty-seven points.

Symptoms of disorders: retention of urine, bed-wetting, delirium, headache, affections of the eye, pain in the meridian area.

The Kidney-Meridian of the Foot—Shaoyin

The kidney-meridian goes from the little toe to its first acupoint on the sole of the foot. It passes the ankle-bone on the inner side, reaches the heel, runs round it and up the leg at the inner end of the knee-flexor fold and up the thigh to the coccyx. It goes on from there to the kidneys, with a ramification to the bladder. It reaches the throat and the root of the tongue via liver, diaphragm and lungs. Its last acupoint is already below the collar-bone. At the level of the lungs there is a ramification to the heart, where the kidney-meridian and the pericardium-meridian join one another.

The kidney-meridian has twenty-seven acupoints.

Symptoms of disorders: hemoptysis, breathlessness, asthma, dryness of the tongue, throat pains or swelling, pains in the back, edema, constipation, diarrhea, weakness of the legs, heat in the soles of the feet, pains in the meridian area.

The Pericardium-Meridian of the Hand—Jueyin

The pericardium-meridian starts in the thorax and goes first to the pericardium, that governs it, then down through the diaphragm into the abdomen, reaching the three levels of the tripartite-warmer one after another. One branch of the meridian leaves the thorax in the neighborhood of the armpit, where its first acupoint is to be found. This branch goes round the armpit and down the inner side of the arm to the elbow flexor-fold, ending in the tip of the middle finger; it occupies the central position among the three Yin-meridians of the hand. A further ramification goes from the palm of the hand to the ring-finger where it links the pericardium-meridian with the tripartite warmer.

The pericardium-meridian has nine acupoints.

The Tripartite Warmer-Meridian of the Hand—Shaoyang

This meridian starts on the ring-finger at the root of the nail and passes between the other two Yang-meridians of the hand over the back of the hand and up the outer side of the arm to the shoulder, where it crosses the gall-bladder-meridian, and then enters the thorax in the hollow over the collar-bone. It meets the pericardium and goes down through the diaphragm to its sponsor, the tripartite warmer. One ramification goes back from the thorax to the collar-bone dip and thence to the neck and round behind the ear to complete its course below the eye-socket. Another ramification enters the ear and surfaces in the direction of the cheek; there it crosses the first ramification and ends in the outward corner of the eye, where it joins the gall-bladder-meridian. There are twenty-three acupoints on this meridian.

Symptoms of disorders: flatulence, bed-wetting, painful urination, deafness, tingling in the ear, throat pains and swellings, pain in the meridian area.

The Gall-Bladder-Meridian of the Foot—Shaoyang

The gall-bladder-meridian runs from the outer corner of the eye via the temples and the ear to the nape of the neck. An initial ramification meets the tripartite warmer-meridian under the eye-socket and runs down into the thorax via the collar-bone hollow. It reaches the abdominal cavity through the diaphragm, joins the liver and approaches the gall-bladder. It then returns to the main meridian at the hip, where the latter has likewise completed its run from the collar-bone down the side of the chest and abdomen. The meridian continues on the outer side of the leg, passes the ankle just above the bone, and comes to an end in the fourth toe. There is a ramification over the instep to the big toe, where it reaches the liver-meridian. We have access to the gall-bladder-meridian at forty-four acupoints.

Symptoms of disorders: a bitter taste in the mouth, dizziness, fever, headache, pains in the upper jaw, inflammation at the outer corner of the eye, deafness, tingling in the ears, pain in the neighborhood of the meridian in general.

The Liver-Meridian of the Foot—Jueyin

The liver-meridian begins in the big toe. It first runs over the instep, passes the ankle in front of the bone on the inner side and crosses the spleen-meridian on its way up the inner side of the shank. Its path continues behind that of the spleen-meridian. In the area of the groin it goes round the genital organs on the outside, rises close to the central body-line through the lower abdomen and then swerves towards the liver, its sponsor, linking both with it and with its Yang partner, the gall-bladder. Reaching the diaphragm, it ceases to be accessible by acupoints and continues to the head, where it joins the eye and ends on the crown. A ramification goes from the eye to the mouth and round it. Another starts in the liver, leaves the abdomen through the diaphragm, joins the lung-meridian in the lung and thus closes the circuit of the twelve regular meridians.

The liver-meridian has fourteen acupoints.

Symptoms of disorders: lumbago, a feeling of oppression in the chest, vomiting, bed-wetting, retention of urine, hernia, pains in the lower abdomen, pains in the area of the meridian.

The Two Special Meridians—Du Mai and Ren Mai

Whereas the regular meridians of the hand and the foot are valid symmetrically for both halves of the body, left and right, and are mutually interchangeable, each with its mirror-image, the eight special meridians enjoy no such duality and have no mirror-image to perform their tasks. Six of them do not even have acupoints of their own but are linked with other meridians at certain points of crossing and junction. They perform co-ordinating functions. The so-called *girdle vessel* (Dai Mai) encircles the waist, collecting the Yin-Yang meridian couples at this central point. Precise knowledge of these special meridians is essential to the specialist, for he must always take into account the various linkage-locations of regular and special meridians when selecting his acupoints for therapy.

Two special meridians also play a central part in self-application of acupressure. The Du Mai and the Ren Mai meridians follow the central body-line, one at the back and the other in the front, making the regular meridians into a co-axial network and offering a large number of valuable acupoints; they do indeed play a central part in every sense of the term.

Du Mai

In Chinese, *mai* is "a vessel," *Du* is "to govern" or "to steer." The main function of this meridian is to steer or govern all the Yang-meridians in the body. It is a Yang-meridian itself, for it rises above the central line of the back, and the back is considered to be Yang from the Chinese point of view. It is often called the "Sea of the Yang-meridians."

Du Mai starts at the perineum and rises via the coccyx and the lumbar vertebrae to the sacrum; there, it first joins the kidneys then continues its route up the spine to the head. It sinks into the brain, rises again to the crown of the head, runs down the middle of the forehead and the nose to the upper lip and ends in the gums above the canines.

Twenty-eight acupoints are directly accessible from the Du Mai meridian.

Symptoms of disorders: feverishness, irritability, stiffness of the spine, tonic spasms of the back-muscles, symptoms of disease in the central nervous system.

Ren Mai

Ren-Mai is the Yin-partner to Du-Mai. *Mai* means "a vessel." *Ren* is "to direct" or "be responsible," the Ren-Mai meridian is responsible for all the Yin-meridians in the body; it is often called "the sea of the Yin meridians." It starts at the perineum, goes up via the pubis, the navel and the breast-bone to the hollow between the under lip and the chin and ends with a circle round the mouth. There are twenty-four acupoints on Ren-Mai.

Symptoms of disorders: Hernia, coughing, asthma, disorders of the urogenital system.

Ren-Mai and Du-Mai, together with the regular meridians, form the system of fourteen classical meridians which constitute the energy supply-network with three hundred and nine acupoints on each body-half and fifty-two on the axial line.

The Acupoints

The system of meridians in the human body is similar to a power-supply network providing energy on a regional basis. In the same way as the power-supply cannot be tapped haphazard but only at established switching-points, the meridians can only be influenced from specific points on their course. These points are the ones we call acupoints. It is in them that the energy gathers and that we can stimulate or stem its flow and regulate its distribution by means of acupressure, acupuncture and moxibustion (heat therapy).

Three hundred and sixty one acupoints have been identified in the course of time. Twenty-eight of these are on the Du Mai-meridian and twenty-four on the Ren Mai-meridian. Since these two meridians follow the central vertical body-line, its axis, one down the back and the other down the chest and abdomen, they are not twinned with a mirror-image, whereas all the other points on the Yin and Yang meridians of hand and foot are presented twice over in the right-hand and left-hand half of the body respectively. It makes no difference to acupress a point on the left or on the right; most of them can be treated on both sides simultaneously. You must remember never to massage an acupoint if the area surrounding it is inflamed; in such cases you only acupress the corresponding point on the other side of the body.

The three hundred and sixty-one acupoints are not all of the same importance. There are some that I use very rarely because the symptoms treated there are highly specific. Others are in constant use because their action regulates the energy flow well beyond their local area. The acupoints below the knee and between the finger-tips and the elbow have always been particularly valuable; the greater the distance from the center of the body, the greater the irregularity of the energy-flow and the easier it becomes to manipulate it with far-reaching effect. Let me illustrate this in a simple way: our hands and feet are the most sensitive and the first to react to the cold; if we rub them, the warmth we produce will pervade and comfort the whole body.

The far-reaching therapeutic action obtainable through acupoints in the extremities was an early discovery. For centuries the old Chinese masters used to say that they could heal every sickness by means of four acupoints. The points they had in mind were the fourth point of the large intestine-meridian on the metacarpus of the forefinger, the thirty-sixth point of the stomach-meridian below the knee, the fortieth point of the bladder-meridian in the hollow of the knee and the seventh point of the lung-meridian above the wrist. These acupoints were described as the four key points of acupuncture. Some physicians used to add the sixth point of the pericardium-meridian and the *Ashi* points, local spots that are painful and sensitive to pressure. Others set aside the *Ashi* points and preferred to take the twenty-sixth point of the Du Mai-meridian.

The twelve Points of Master Ma

About 960 under the Song dynasty, Master Ma recommended the use of twelve acupoints, which to his mind contained all the therapeutic indications and action-potential of the three hundred and fifty-seven acupoints that were known at that time. Together with the four key points, his list included the following: the forty-fourth point of the stomach-meridian, the eleventh point of the large intestine-meridian, the third point of the liver-meridian, the thirtieth and the thirty-fourth point of the gall-bladder-meridian, the fifth point of the heart-meridian, the fifty-seventh and the sixtieth points of the bladder-meridian. Therapy possibilities for acupuncture using these twelve points are indeed manifold, as you may see from the following indications for treatment: *stomach-meridian 36 (Zusanti)*: disorders of the digestive tract, gastrospasms, nausea and vomiting, flatulence, constipation, dysentery, enteritis. This acupoint can be used to brace up the whole system.

large intestine meridian 4 (Hegu): headache, toothache, catarrh, tonsilitis, pharyngitis, ophtalmodynia, paralysis of the facial muscles, goiter, pain and paralysis in the upper extremities, excessive and deficient sweat secretion, chills, fever.

bladder-meridian 40 (Weizhong): sciatica, pains in the back, paralysis of the lower extremities, sunburn, affections of the knee.

Lung-meridian 7 (Lieque): headache, stiff neck, cough, asthma, paralysis of the facial muscles, trigeminal neuralgia.

stomach-meridian 44 (Neiting): stomach pains, headache, toothache, tonsilitis, dysentery.

large intestine-meridian 11 (Guchi): pains in the arm or shoulder, paralysis of the upper limbs, affections of the elbow, fever, eczema, high blood-pressure.

gall-bladder-meridian 30 (Huantiao): paralysis of the lower limbs, affections of the hip.

gall-bladder-meridian 34 (Yanglingquan): hemiplegia, affections of the bile ducts, pains in the back and legs.

heart-meridian 5 (Tongli): headache, acute hoarseness, stiffness of the tongue, speech defects, insomnia, palpitations, pains in the arm and wrist.

liver-meridian 3 (Taichong): headache, giddiness, epilepsy, feverish convulsions in children, diseases of the eye, hernia, metrorrhagia as apart from menstruation, mastitis.

bladder-meridian 60 (Kunlun): paralysis of the lower limbs, pains in the back, sciatica, pains in the joints.

bladder-meridian 57 (Chengshan): sciatica, intestinal prolapse, cramp in the calves, pain in the sole of the foot, paralysis of the lower limbs.

Note on the inter-relationship of the meridians as shown in the illustration:—The lung-meridian links with the liver-meridian and the large-intestine-meridian. Two meridians, one pertaining to the hand and the other to the foot, are covered by the same term. The lung-, heart- and pericardium-meridians are the three Yin meridians of the hand that run outwards, viz. from the body to the extremities.

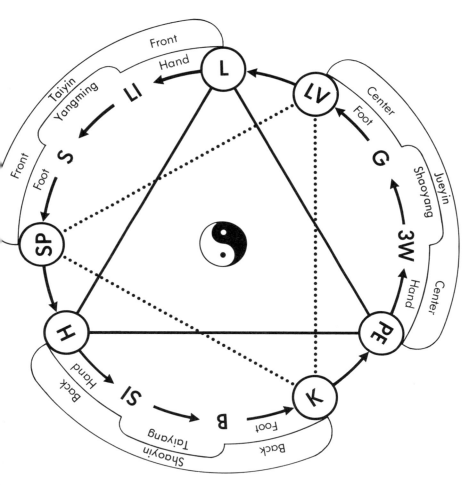

3 Yang-meridians [of] the hand [run] inwards	3 Yin-meridians of the hand run outwards	3 Yang-meridians of the foot run outwards	3 Yin-meridians of the foot run inwards

L lung-meridian of the hand—Taiyin	B bladder-meridian of the foot—Taiyang
LI large intestine-meridian of the hand—Yangming	K kidney-meridian of the foot—Shaoyin
S Stomach-meridian of the foot—Yangming	PE pericardium-meridian of hand—Jueyin
SP spleen-meridian of the foot—Taiyin	3W tripartite warmer-meridian of the hand—Shaoyang
H heart-meridian of the hand—Shaoyin	G gall-bladder-meridian of the foot—Shaoyang
SI small intestine-meridian of the hand—Taiyang	LV liver-meridian of the foot—Jueyin

Cun—Your Personal Yardstick

The fact that our body measurements vary considerably from one person to another used to be a frequent cause of error when locating acupoints on an individual patient. Some two thousand years ago, under the Han dynasty, the doctors decided to take all measurements individually on the basis of a unit they called *Cun* (Tchun), the breadth of the human thumb, which had been found to constitute a personal constant.

One Cun is the breadth of your thumb. The breadth of the four remaining fingers placed side by side together is equal to three Cun. Two fingers are a Cun and a half. Cun as a yardstick could not be simpler; it provides a convenient means to locate acupoints, particularly for persons doing their own acupressure without outside assistance. One must bear in mind however that the breadth of the fingers may be affected by occupational activities. The following list shows the main proportional body measurements, so you can check and see whether your personal cun is in line with the indications given.

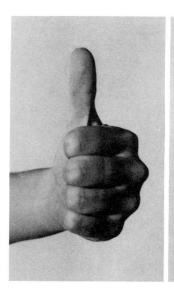
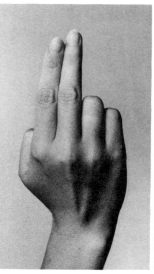
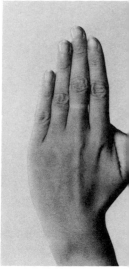

Head

12 cun:
    the scalp, from the forehead to the nape of the neck.

3 cun: the central point between the eyebrows to the edge of the scalp.

3 cun: the edge of the scalp in the nape of the neck to the seventh vertebra, easily found on account of its prominence.

Trunk

8 cun: the distance between the nipples.

8 cun: from the navel to the sternum.

5 cun: from the navel to the pubis.

6 cun: between the two inside edges of the shoulder-blades.

Arms

9 cun: from the front end of the armpit fold to the crook of the arm.

12 cun: from the crook of the arm to the wrist flexor.

Legs

19 cun: from the greater trochanter to the center of the knee-cap.

16 cun: from the center of the knee-cap to the outer edge of the ankle.

There are two different ways in which you can locate acupoints: either by using the breadth of the thumb as equal to one cun or by referring to proportional measurements, where the distances between two obvious points are broken down into a standard number of cun units. You can find a point that lies two cun above the wrist by measuring the breadth of your thumb twice over. You can also locate it by dividing the distance from your wrist to the crook of the arm into twelve equal parts (12 cun) with a tape-measure and pressing the point at the end of the second section above the wrist. The second method is more accurate, although not quite so simple; I should think the direct measurement in finger-breadths is adequate when doing acupressure by yourself. After all, the proportional method of measurement is also an approximation; it can only help you to locate the acupoint in a general way. It is the sensitivity of the relevant point that will show you whether you have really found it. Under a constant pressure, the reaction of an acupoint is much more marked than that of any other spot in the vicinity. So you should feel for the most sensitive spot in a wider area. There is another peculiarity of acupoints that will help you: most of them lie in hollow places that are not visible to the naked eye but can be immediately perceived by the fingers.

Practical Application

Whether the acupoints are to be treated traditionally with gold and silver needles, or by ultra-modern Laser-techniques, or with one's bare hands, the purpose of the therapy remains unchanged: it is to regulate the energy flow, to restore the balance of Yin and Yang in the human organism. The first-named techniques are more precise and therefore more effective than acupressure, but they are also more dangerous unless they are perfectly mastered by the specialist. There are even risks in acupressure. For instance, pressure with the finger-nails increases precision, but it also increases the risk of infection if the skin is injured in any way; the finger-nails are not aseptic like the acupuncteur's needles. I recommend using the finger-tips—forefinger or thumb are best—or the ball of the thumb for massage. Then you really can't go wrong and will be able to apply your own acupressure safely. The method has a further practical advantage: whereas the acupuncture needles must hit the target with absolute precision, the relatively large area treated by hand is bound to include the target as well. So, do not dispair if you try to cure some ailment mentioned in this book by means of acupressure and find you do not succeed straight away. I have been practising for many years and have found that most people are able to learn acupressure; as time passes you will find it increasingly easy to locate the acupoints precisely and to distinguish their degree of sensitivity from that of other parts of the relevant area.

Professional acupressers combine various forms of massage according to the purpose of the therapy. You have for instance "pulling," "rubbing," "knocking," "pushing," "pressing at one point," "pressing with a circular motion." The last-named technique is particularly suitable when applying acupressure to yourself. If you acupress clockwise and anti-clockwise in turn, you will be applying the equalizing principle of Yin and Yang. When you massage clockwise you are giving Yang, anti-clockwise you are counter-balancing Yang with Yin. The body will automatically take in more of the energy that it needs. The pressure exerted should be at least strong enough to move the tissue with the finger circling over it.

In the illustrated section of the book, you will see that I make a distinction between *main points* ●, and *secondary points*, ○. This is not a quality assessment. It does not mean that some points are less important than others. You should massage all the points that are mentioned in respect of a given ailment. The "main points" are however the ones you must massage a little longer and more frequently than the "secondary'' ones, so that their effect, specific to the ailment, may develop fully.

Acupress the points indicated, in any order, until you feel some relief. The treatment can be repeated several times in one day, but do not acupress for more than twenty to twenty-five minutes at a time.

If there is no improvement, do not put off seeing your doctor. You can still go on using acupressure—particularly if you are in pain—as a transitional therapy while you are waiting for an appointment. Why remain inactive if you have the means to do something for yourself!

In compiling this section, I have tried to restrict myself to common every-day complaints: either such ailments as a cold in the head, which do not usually mean a visit to the doctor for an otherwise healthy person, or chronic disorders such

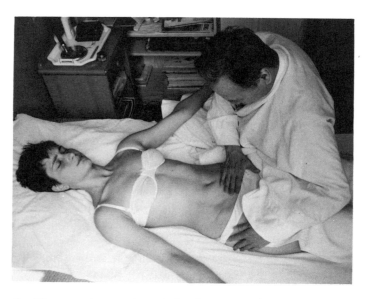

Dr. Hin massaging a patient; the hands move gently over the body, loosening tension, setting the body fluids flowing, restoring the energy-balance.

as arthritis, where conventional medicine still has little to offer beyond analgesics for external or internal use.

In the following cases, you should consult your doctor before having recourse to acupressure therapy:

– if you are undergoing medical treatment for any complaint;
– if you suffer from high blood-pressure;
– during pregnancy.

The old Chinese masters were able to heal disease without physical contact with the patient: they concentrated on the relevant acupoints and set their energy flowing. Times have changed and this degree of perfection is now beyond us. All I have been able to achieve so far is to apply mental acupressure to myself and to obtain the same beneficial effects as by physical action.

NERVOSITY

Sometimes we know why our nerves are on edge: an examination, a new job, a journey, an important festivity may reduce us to such a state of excitement that we can neither eat nor sleep and our hearts beat wildly at the mere thought of these events. Fear, incertitude and anticipation are among the most frequent causes of nervosity.

Nervosity becomes a health problem when it has no apparent cause, but develops into a permanent condition, causing distress to the sufferer and to those who associate with him. A couple can hardly enjoy a pleasant evening together if one of them has a fit of nerves whenever their baby cries. The parents may even start quarreling and the baby will react by beginning to cry again. In this case it is not the baby's fault and it is up to the parents to "keep their cool" and restrain themselves. Even if the child still cries they will probably notice it less; in all probability it will indeed cry far less frequently once it feels that its parents are present and in harmony.

This applies in various circumstances. We should think less of "making the baby stop crying" and more of strengthening our minds and learning to retain our composure in spite of incidental aggression of the nervous system. Acupressure can help us. Since nervosity is seldom due to organic causes, we shall have recourse in the first place to those acupoints in the extremities whose therapeutic action extends far beyond their local area.

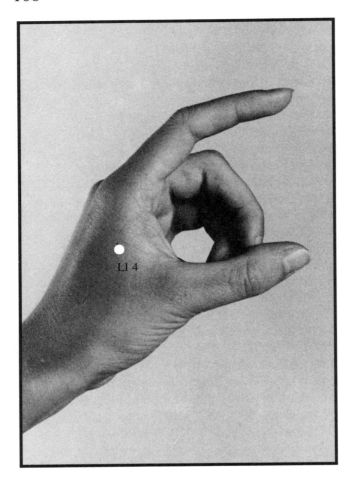

LI 4

You will find *LI 4* of the large intestine-meridian, one of the oldest acupoints in Chinese medicine, on the metacarpus of the forefinger. If you flatten your hand and press the thumb against it, there will be a small hillock on the back of the hand. Put your other thumb on the top of it and relax the hand. This is the point you want.

SP 6 of the spleen-meridian (Sanyinjiao, meeting of the three Yin) lies three cun above the ankle-bone. You will find it easier to operate with your foot on the other knee. (Top left, opposite page 109)

LV 3 of the Liver-meridian is two cun below the space between the big toe and second toe, (bottom left, opposite page 109)

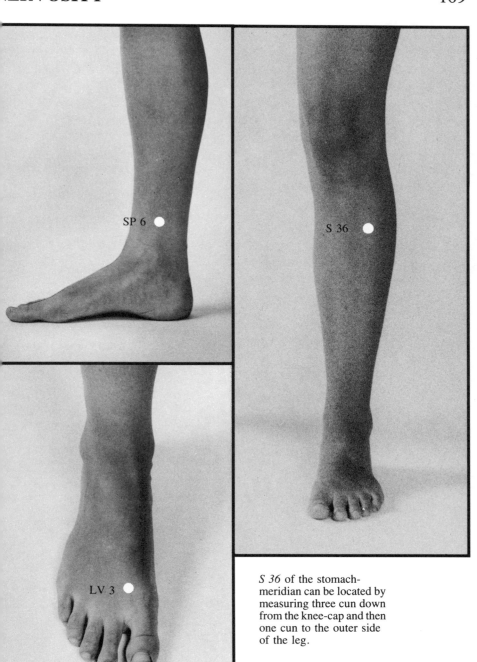

S 36 of the stomach-meridian can be located by measuring three cun down from the knee-cap and then one cun to the outer side of the leg.

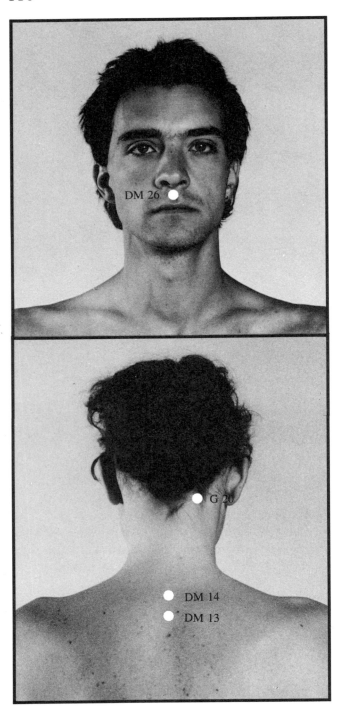

DM 26 of the Du Mai-meridian lies two-thirds of the distance from the upper lip to the nose.

DM 13 of the Du Mai-meridian lies below the first thoracic vertebra.

DM 14 of the Du Mai-meridian lies below the seventh cervical vertebra. This vertebra sticks out more than the others when you bow your head. *G20* of the gall-bladder-meridian is located between two muscles and easy to feel if you bow your head and move it from side to side.

PALPITATIONS

In China, the heart is considered to be the seat of the mind. Since our health is influenced essentially by our state of mind, we have to take very great care of it and of the organ wherein it resides. In Chinese medicine, strengthening the mind is a priority for every therapy; its good health is the primary precondition even for the healing of a harmless flesh-wound. In the Western world, where so many people's lives—both at work and play—are dominated by time-frames and deadlines, the heart and mind are subjected to pretty rough treatment. It is no wonder that more and more people feel that they are doing too much, although most of them fail to admit it, even to themselves. This leads to situations of stress and an ever widening gap between the expectations of society and people's awareness of their own limited capabilities. The result may be anxiety, anguish, depression; if things come to the worst, the heart may fail.

Anxiety and palpitations often go together. By strengthening the heart, we are strengthening the spirit, weakened by fear, and my therapy therefore concentrates primarily on the acu-points of the heart- and the pericardium-meridians and action through them. A further point I use stimulates the Bladder-meridian, for this meridian is linked by the Chinese element "Water" with the emotion of fear.

Palpitations of the heart may be due to fear and they can also be its origin. So try to distinguish clearly between cause and effect. Your palpitations may also be the result of some physical disorder which should be explored by the doctor.

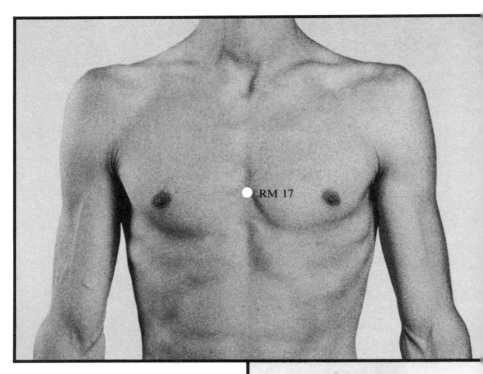

RM 17 of the Ren Mai-meridian is on the sternum in the exact center of the chest between the nipples; it is called Shanzhong. You locate it when lying down, for the nipples will then be in their anatomically correct position in the fourth inter-costal space.

H 7 of the heart-meridian is on the wrist fold, outside the line connecting wrist and elbow. If you measure two cun up the arm from the center of the fold, you reach *PE 6* of the pericardium-meridian, which is called the ''inner link'' (Neiguan).

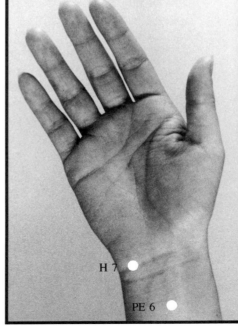

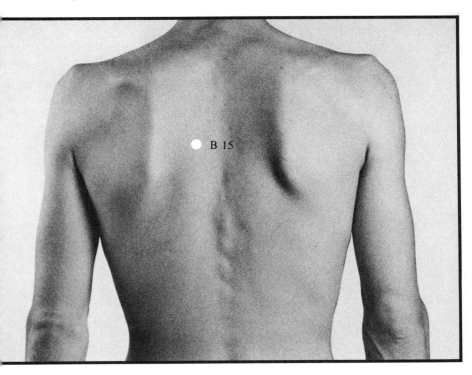

You may need somebody else's assistance to locate and acupress *B 15* of the bladder-meridian. It will be easier for your partner if you bend your back. The point is one and a half cun to the side of the fifth thoracic vertebra and can be located by counting from the lowest cervical vertebra, which stands out when you bend your head.

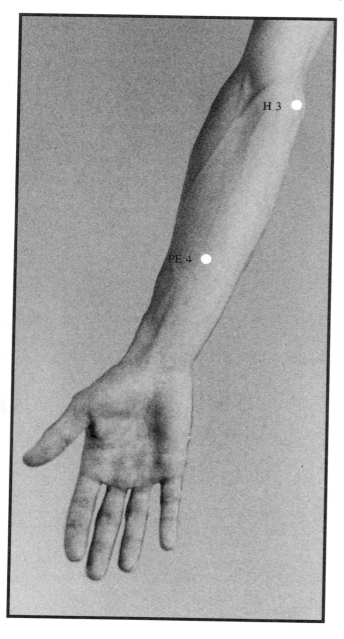

When you bend your arm t
form a right angle, *H 3* of
the heart-meridian will be a
the end of the fold nearest t
body. *PE 4* of the
pericardium-meridian is in t
middle of the arm, on the inn
side, exactly five cun above
the wrist-fold.

DEPRESSION

Surely we all know those gloomy days, dark and bleak as November, days when we know as soon as we wake in the morning that the clouds will not lift . . .

Some people will put this down to a hitch in their biodynamics. Others may see it in the light of an uneven struggle between their It, their Ego and their super-Ego. Others again will seek relief in a cigarette and a pick-me-up with their morning coffee. Finally there are some people who will simply telephone their work-place to say that they are ill and stay safely in their beds with their eyes shut. However varied our behavioral approach to the gloomy days, they are always times when we feel weary, out of sorts, with no desire to do anything or see anybody.

Frequently these states of depression are not due to anything we can put our finger on. The conclusions reached in Chinese medicine may even seem a little strange to the Western reader. They are only comprehensible if you remember that the physical and the spiritual, body and soul, are considered as an inseparable entity. The spirit dwells in the heart. If the heart is undernourished or incorrectly nourished, the spirit may withdraw, leaving a void of which we are only too aware in our apathy and absence of desire. Our therapy to overcome these characteristic Yin symptoms is by stimulating acupoints on the heart-meridian, on the pericardium-meridian close-by and on the spleen-meridian which is directly linked to that of the heart. In addition, we massage a number of powerful acupoints on the Yang meridians of the stomach, the gall-bladder and the Du Mai.

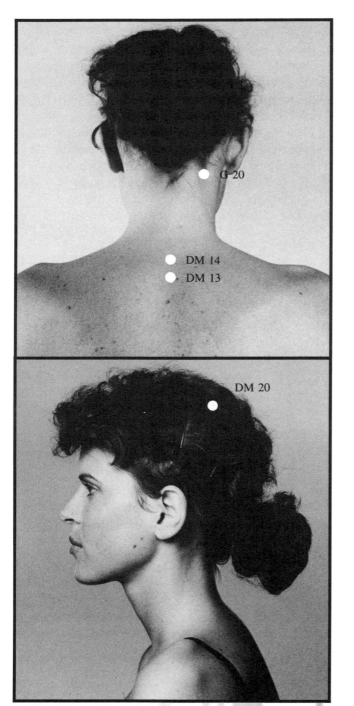

Du Mai-meridian 13, *DM 13*, is a point just below the first thoracic vertebra. *DM 14* is just below the seventh cervical vertebra. *G 20* of the gall-bladder-meridian lies in the hollow just across the first muscle from the root of the hair, that is called "the windy pool" (*Fengchi*).

If you start from the central point between your eyebrows and measure eight cun, viz. twice the breadth of your thumb and twice the breadth of your hand, over your forehead and the crown of your head, you will come to *DM 20* of the Du Mai-meridian, called the "place of one hundred concordances" (*Baihui*).

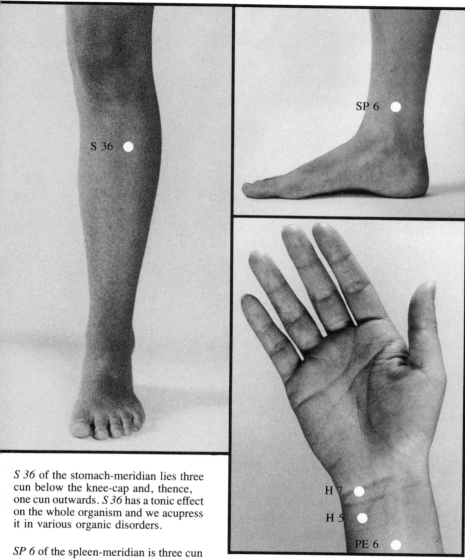

S 36 of the stomach-meridian lies three cun below the knee-cap and, thence, one cun outwards. S 36 has a tonic effect on the whole organism and we acupress it in various organic disorders.

SP 6 of the spleen-meridian is three cun above the ankle-bone on the inner side. It is the point where the spleen-meridian meets the other two Yin meridians of the foot, which are the Liver- and the Kidney-meridian; it is called Sanyinjiao—"the meeting of the three Yin."

H 5 of the heart-meridian—called Tongli—"interior understanding"— lies one cun away from H 7, "the Gate of the spirit" (Shenmen); both of these are of major importance when treating depression. Two cun away from the wrist-fold where we located H 7, we shall find PE 6 of the pericardium-meridian in the central area of the forearm.

INSOMNIA

Soporifics, together with analgesics, stimulants and sedatives, all come under the heading *hypnotica*. Their side-effects may be physically or psychically dangerous. An over-dose may lead to a fatal issue. Prolonged, regular use creates dependency. Old people often suffer from a number of organic troubles that cause insomnia and there may be mental and emotional problems into the bargain. Loneliness, inactivity, reduced autonomy, doubts as to the purpose of life, fear of death—all these things make it increasingly difficult to get to sleep and for many elderly people the sleeping-pill becomes part of their bedtime routine.

Particularly for these older people, who may be having to take various drugs in any case, acupressure, which has no side-effects for them to worry about, may prove to be of valuable assistance. The main acupoints are heart-meridian 7 and pericardium-meridian 6, both located on the wrist and easy to acupress, even for people who are handicapped in their movements.

You must take insomnia seriously! It could be a symptom of organic or psychic trouble that requires treatment by a physician. You still should begin by exploring the problem yourself and trying to discover its origin and find a solution. Perhaps it is too hot in your bedroom, or there may be light or noise from the street? Perhaps you drink too much tea or coffee or alcohol? Are you taking some drug or home remedy that might interfere with your night's rest? Are you doing too much, either in your job or at home? Do you spend too much time watching television? Acupressure cannot remove the cause, whatever it may be, but it will certainly help you to get to sleep if you acupress the points indicated, regularly and gently.

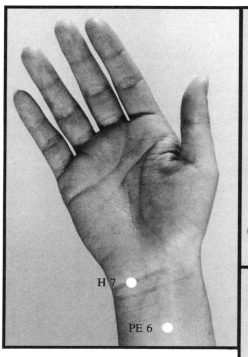

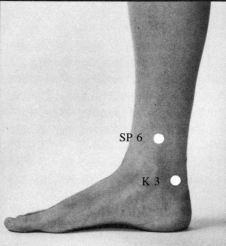

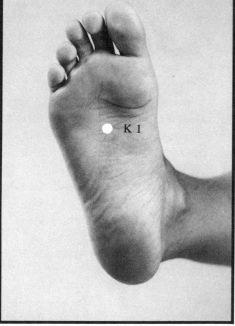

H 7 of the heart-meridian is called
Shenmen, "the gate of the spirit." It
is on the outer end of wrist fold, at
one side of the ligament running from
wrist to elbow. *PE 6* of the pericardium-
meridian is two cun away from the first
wrist-fold, up the arm.

SP 6 of the spleen-meridian is three cun
above the ankle-bone. *K 3* of the kidney-
meridian is in the hollow between the
tip of the ankle-bone and the Achilles'
tendon. Move your finger back
horizontally from the bone to avoid
pressing *K 4* by mistake—only half a
cun below *K 3!*

You cannot miss *K 1* of the kidney-
meridian if you feel for a hollow spot
in the sole of the foot, two-thirds of
its length as from the heel end.

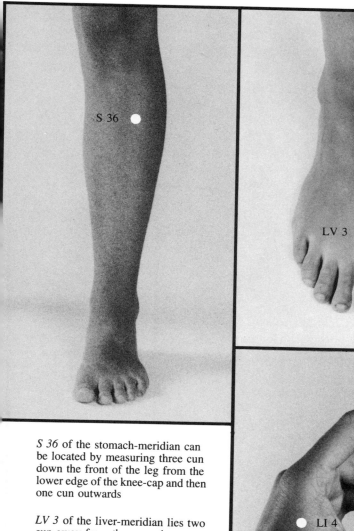

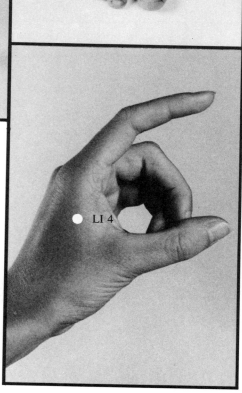

S 36 of the stomach-meridian can be located by measuring three cun down the front of the leg from the lower edge of the knee-cap and then one cun outwards

LV 3 of the liver-meridian lies two cun away from the space between the big toe and the second toe. It is called *Taichong*—"flood-tide"

LI 4 of the large intestine-meridian is called *Hegu*—"the enclosed valley." You locate the point by pressing your thumb against the metacarpus so that a small hillock appears on the back of the hand. Put your finger on the top of this and acupress it after relaxing the hand.

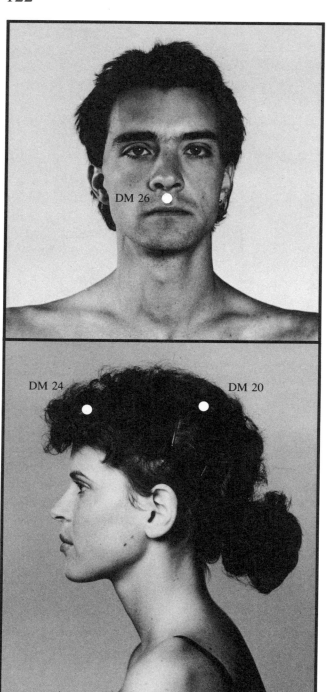

DM 26 of the Du Mai-meridian is located between the nose and the upper lip, two-thirds above the lip, in the middle.

DM 24 is half a cun above the roots of the hair; it can be located by measuring three and a half cun above the centerpoint between the eyebrows. Eight cun further over the crown takes you to *DM 20* of the same Du Mai-meridian.

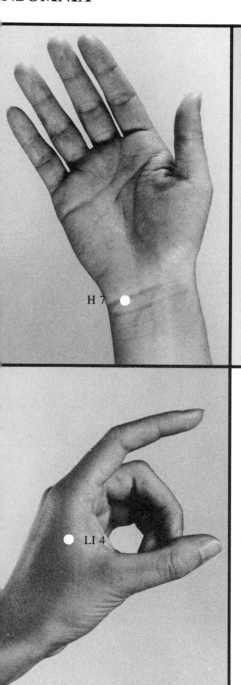

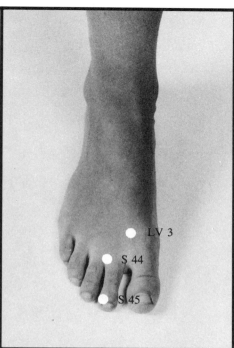

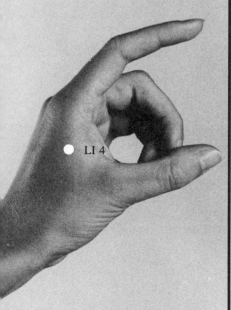

H 7 of the heart-meridian lies on the outer side of the ligament connecting ulna and wrist. It is called *Shenmen,* "the gate of the spirit."

LV 3 of the liver-meridian, called *Taichong,* "the flood-tide," lies two cun away from the space between the big toe and the second toe. *S 44* of the stomach-meridian, called *Neitang,* "the inner court," is half a cun away from the space between the second and third toe. *S 45*, the final point of the stomach-meridian, is on the outer corner of the nail of the second toe.

LI 4 of the large intestine-meridian is located by putting your finger on the small hillock that appears on the other hand when you press the thumb against the metacarpus. You acupress, after relaxing the hand.

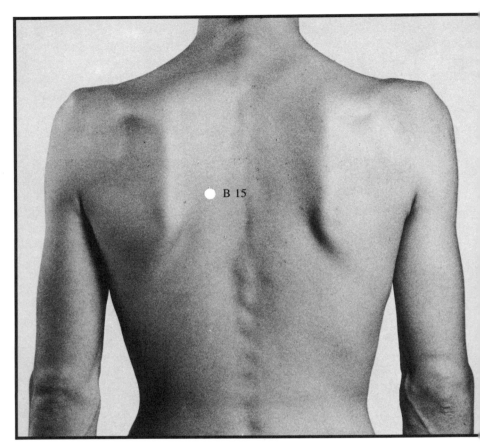

Acupressure on *B 15* of the bladder-
meridian will probably require outside
assistance. It is located one and a half
cun to the side of the spinous process
of the fifth thoracic vertebra.

HEADACHE

It may be a shooting, burning, throbbing pain, it may feel like a hammering, a heavy weight, a dull oppression. Few ailments make themselves felt in so many different ways and are frequently as hard to describe as a headache. And yet every headache is a symptom. It may be due to a cerebral tumor, to neurological disorders, or to facial ones, particularly those of the eyes. Many women complain of headache during menstruation, or at the time of the menopause. The causes may be psychic. It may be due to high blood-pressure. The exhaust-pipe of your vehicle may be faulty. There may be toxic fumes at your work-place. It may come from something very simple like bad posture. Chinese medicine also relates headache to perturbations of the energy flow on specific meridians: pain in the forehead concerns the stomach-meridian, pain in the temples the gall-bladder-meridian, pain in the back of the head and the crown of the head concern the bladder- and the liver-meridian respectively.

In all cases of headache, acupressure is an obvious and ideal form of therapy. Unlike pain-killers, it has no side-effects. Sometimes the mere relaxation of posture acupressing entails may bring relief.

Together with local points on the head, we acupress exclusively the so-called "distant points," viz. beyond the elbow and below the knee, which have a specific analgesic effect on distant parts of the anatomy. You should always try to relax completely, mentally and physically, before you start acupressure. The more relaxed you are, the sooner you may expect results.

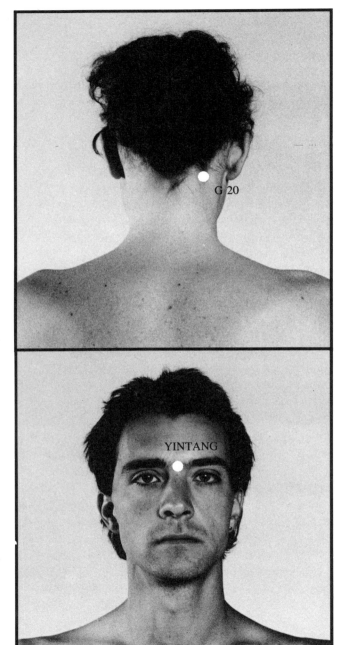

G 20 of the gall-bladder-meridian lies in a hollow beside the trapeze muscle at the root of the hair. It is called *Fenchi,* ''The windy pool,'' and is a main acupoint for pain in the whole head.

FOREHEAD
Yintang lies in the center between the eyebrows. It is a ''special point'' and is on the same line as the Du Mai-meridian, but it does not belong to it.

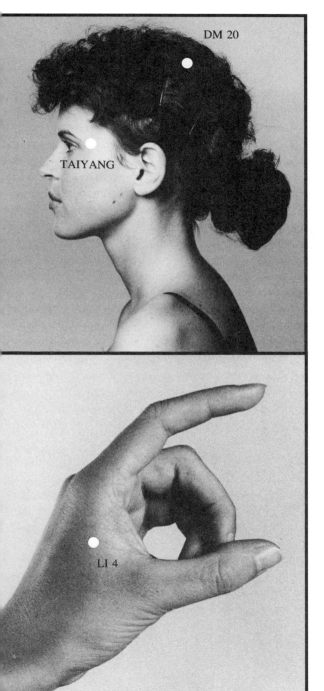

DM 20

TAIYANG

LI 4

HEADACHE (TEMPLES)

Taiyang, another "special point" not belonging to any meridian, is between the outer corner of the eye and the eyebrow, one cum outwards. *DM 20* of the Du Mai-meridian is measured from the central point between the eyebrows, eight cun up and over the crown of the head.

LI 4 of the large intestine-meridian is located by putting your finger on the top of the small hillock that appears when you press your thumb against the metacarpus of the hand. You acupress after relaxing the hand.

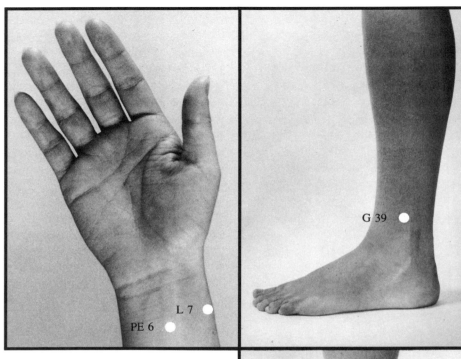

PE 6 of the pericardium-meridian is in
the center of the forearm, on the inner
side, two cun from the first wrist-fold.
L 7 of the lung-meridian is a cun and
a half beyond the joint of the wrist and
is the point you touch with the tip of
your forefinger if you cross your thumbs
so that the fingers rest on the upper side
of the hand and wrist.

G 39 of the gall-bladder-meridian,
called Xuanzhong, ''the swinging bell''
is three cun above the ankle-bone on
the outer side.

S 44 of the stomach-meridian is half a
cun from the space between the second
and third toe.

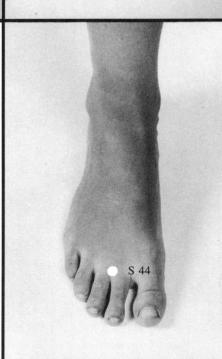

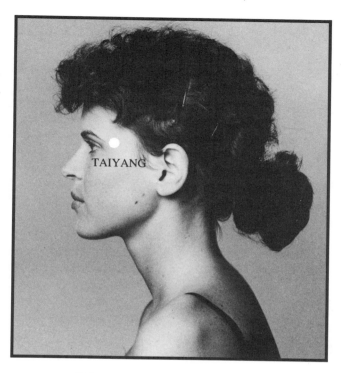

Taiyang, a special point outside the meridians, is located by measuring one cun outwards from the center between the outer corner of the eye and the eyebrow.

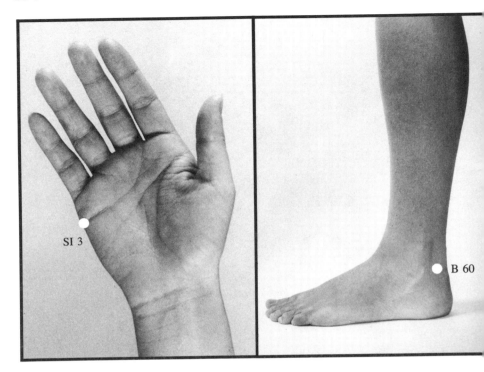

The palm of the hand is well irrigated and darker in color than the other side; this color demarcation-line is visible from the side; *SI 3* of the small intestine-meridian is on this line, below the little finger.

B 60 of the bladder-meridian is in the hollow between the ankle-bone and the Achilles-tendon, on the outer side.

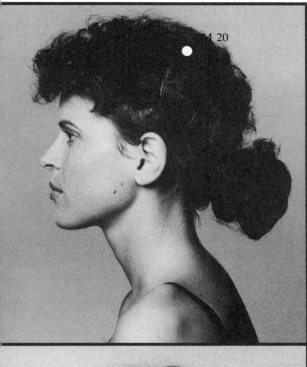

DM 20 of the Du Mai-meridian is the main acupoint for pain in the top of the head. It is called *Baihui*, "the place of the one hundred concordances." Measure eight cun over the head from the center between the eyebrows.

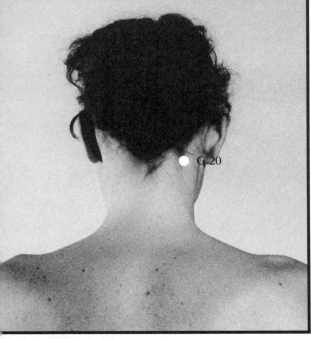

G 20 of the gall-bladder-meridian, called *Fenchi*, "the windy pool," is in the hollow beside the trapeze, which is the muscle going up the nape of the neck on either side of the cervical vertebrae; one can feel it by moving your head from side to side.

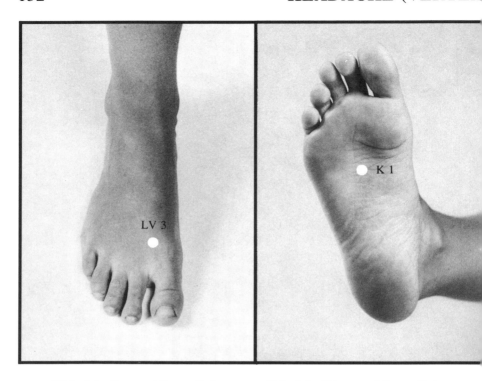

LV 3 of the liver-meridian, called "flood-tide," *Taichong,* is in the inter-tarsal space, two cun away from the big toe and the second toe. We again stress that it is from the "distant points," located in the extremities (below the knee or the elbow), that we can treat far-away areas of the anatomy.

K 1 of the kidney-meridian, called *Yangquan,* "the gushing spring," is in the sole of the foot, two-thirds of the distance from the heel.

DEBILITY

There are two main acupoints for the treatment of debility and failing strength. One is *RM 4* on the Ren Mai-meridian, called *Guanyuan*, "the pivot of life," which is described in our textbooks as a point of tonification for the whole organism. The other has similar virtues and is *S 36* on the stomach-meridian; in ancient times, the Chinese foot-soldiers pressed it on their long weary marches.

Chinese diagnostics consider weariness and feelings of weakness to be signs of emptiness, a void. They are usually a sign of low blood-pressure. People with low blood-pressure frequently complain that they "see stars" when they stoop down, or that everything "goes black" when they have to lift something heavy. They feel weak, as though they had lost blood, some of them lose consciousness. Acupressure can stabilize the blood-pressure and prevent a sudden drop in particular circumstances.

Blood-pressure that tends to be low is not usually a danger to the health, but we should do something about it nevertheless. It may cause lassitude of the mind as well as the body. We find it hard to concentrate, lose the thread of a conversation, forget what a newspaper-article is about before we have read to the end. These symptoms too can be overcome with the help of acupressure.

A balanced diet, rich in vitamins, will prove an effective adjuvant to the acupressure therapy. Biological special products like pollen are also most helpful in cases of low blood-pressure.

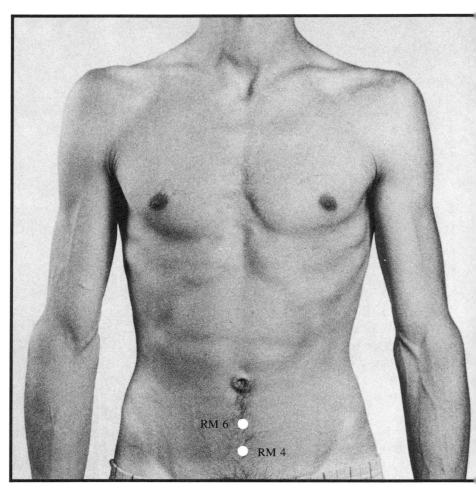

RM 4 and *RM 6* of the Ren Mai-meridian are on the axle of the abdomen. *RM 6,* called *Qihai,* ''the sea of energy,'' is one cun and a half below the navel. *RM 4,* called *Guanyuan,* ''the pivot of life,'' is located a further cun and a half down.

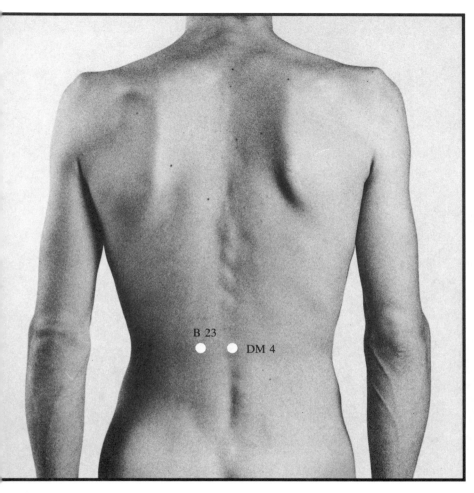

B 23 of the bladder-meridian and *DM 4* of the Du Mai-meridian are approached in the small of the back. Going round the waist on the level of the navel, you find *DM 4*, called *Mingmen*, ''the gate of life,'' between the spinous processes of the second and third lumbar vertebrae, and *B 23* beside it, a cun and a half further on.

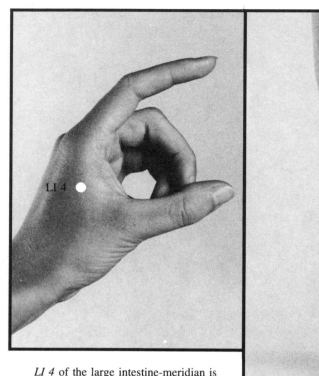

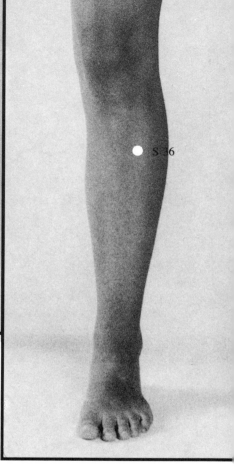

LI 4 of the large intestine-meridian is called *Hegu,* "the enclosed valley." You locate it by putting your finger on top of the small hillock that appears when you press the thumb of the other hand against the metacarpus and acupress after relaxing the hand.

S 36 of the stomach-meridian lies three cun down the front of the leg from the lower edge of the knee-cap, then one cun outwards. It is a point of overall tonification.

VERTIGO

A little while ago, a prosperous-looking Lebanese gentleman came to consult me, complaining that he frequently felt dizzy. I noticed that he seemed to be somewhat nervy and on edge. I listened while he described his trouble and then cautiously asked about his circumstances in general, his family, his profession. He said he was a business-man, he was married and his four grown-up children were studying in Paris. He and his wife travelled continually; she had a shop for office-equipment in Africa. The more I listened the more convinced I became that his trouble was not vertigo but his nerves. I gave him acupuncture on that basis. A few days later he came back, highly delighted and accompanied by his wife. He assured me that the dizziness was gone. I gave him the same therapy as before and after I had placed the needles I went to talk to his wife in the next room. She confirmed my diagnosis. Her husband's nerves had been in such a condition that he could not bear the sound of turning the pages of a book if she ever started reading in bed.

So the origin of that case of dizziness was clearly psychic; and that indeed is quite frequent, although it does not mean that there are not physical causes of vertigo as well. Often it is due to eye trouble, or irritation of the internal ear, where our sense of balance is centered.

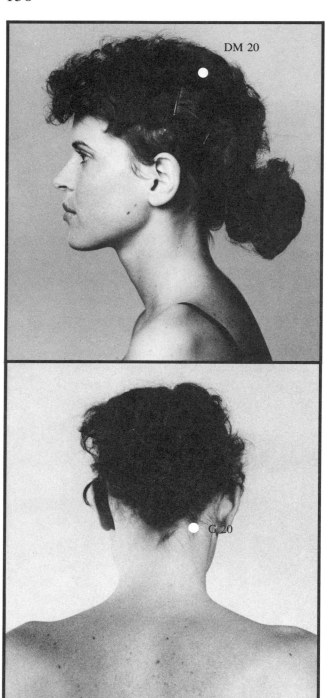

DM 20 of the Du Mai-meridian is measured from the central point between the eyebrows and eight cur up over the vertex, the crown of the head. This point is called *Baihu*i, "the place of one hundred concordances."

G 20 of the gall-bladder-meridian lies in a hollow beside the trapeze muscle, which goes up the nape of the neck on either side of the cervical vertebrae.

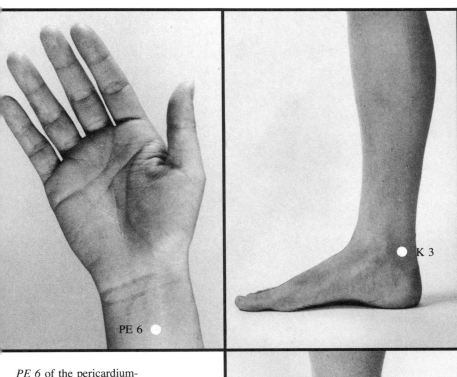

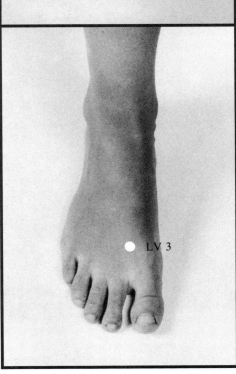

PE 6 of the pericardium-meridian is in the center of the forearm, two cun from the first wrist-fold. It is called *Neiguan*, ''the inner link.''

K 3 of the kidney-meridian is in the hollow between the ankle-bone and the Achilles-tendon on the same level as the bone.

LV 3 of the liver-meridian lies between the big toe and the second toe, two cun away.

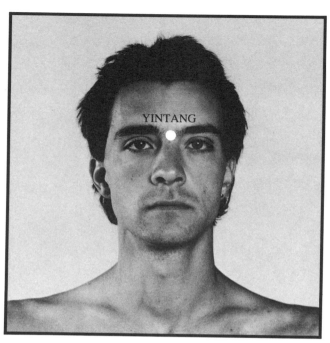

Yintang is a special point and lies in
the center between the eyebrows.

HOW TO STOP SMOKING

It is now common knowledge that smoking constitutes a major risk as regards the contraction of various diseases. Already in the 'Sixties scientists had been able to calculate the precise degree of probability for smokers to be affected as compared to non-smokers: in the case of lung-cancer with a fatal issue the risk for smokers is 10.8 times greater than for non-smokers of the same age; in the case of bronchitis and emphysema it is 6.1 times greater; in the case of laringeal or thyroid cancer it is 5.4 times greater. These are all scientific findings and one can hardly say that the area has not been properly explored.

It certainly takes will-power to stop yourself from smoking, although that in itself is not always enough. Some people actually decide to stop smoking and do stop smoking overnight. Others have the same intention and do their best with anti-nicotine chewing-gum, detoxication filters, or press-studs in the ear. I have had to treat a great many nicotine addicts and I have noticed an interesting point: patients who are preponderantly Yin—people whose blood-pressure is low, who feel the cold and like hot drinks and hot food—are usually the ones who find it most difficult to give up smoking. Unconsciously, they are seeking in their cigarette the Yang element of fire and its vitalizing warmth.

Acupressure can help you to resist your craving for a smoke. This is particularly important during the first few days of deprivation. Use acupressure to strengthen your will and evade psychic side-effects during weaning by using the acupoints for DEPRESSION and NERVOSITY in addition to those given specifically in this chapter.

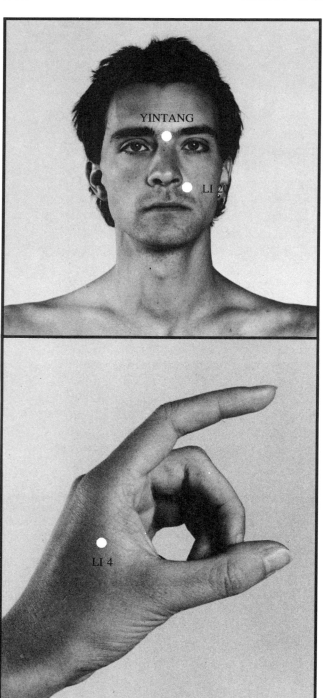

Yintang is a special point that was discovered later than those of the classical meridian-system. It is centrally located between the eyebrows. *LI 20* of the large intestine-meridian lies between the nostril and the line running down from the nose to the corner of the mouth.

LI 4 of the large intestine-meridian is located by putting your finger on the little hillock that appears on the other hand when you press its thumb against it. Acupress after relaxing the hand.

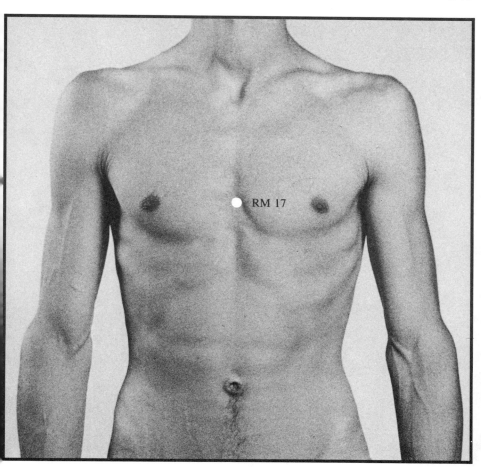

RM 17 of the Ren Mai meridian lies in the center between the nipples and is best located when lying down so that the nipples are in their correct anatomical position on the level of the fourth intercostal space.

PAIN

"Chinese traditional medicine and pharmaceutica are a rich inheritance; we must explore them with renewed diligence and pursue their development to a high level"; those were the words of President Mao in person. In the late 'Fifties Chinese physicians had already produced spectacular findings that soon received world-wide attention. It was on the basis of our age-old knowledge of the analgesic action of acupuncture that they developed acupuncture-anesthesia. Twenty years later there had already been more than a hundred successful open-heart operations in which the patients had remained fully conscious during surgery and had survived without having to suffer the after-effects of long narcosis. The advantages of acupuncture-anesthesia are obvious: narcosis risks are eliminated, the patient is conscious and can contribute personally to the success of the operation and he will get well again sooner because his physiological functions have hardly been restricted at all while the operation was going on.

The purpose of the above digression was to stress the power of acupuncture to relieve pain; I wanted to encourage you to have recourse to it in less drastic circumstances than those I described. There is no area in which the success of Chinese medicine has been more readily recognized than in that of analgesia.

Acupressure, as a "gentler version" of acupuncture," can likewise relieve pain whatever its cause—arthrosis, injury, or constriction of a nerve. If the pain is of an arthritic nature, you can combine arthritic points with local ones, taking care not to massage the affected joint, but the one corresponding to it on the other side of your anatomy.

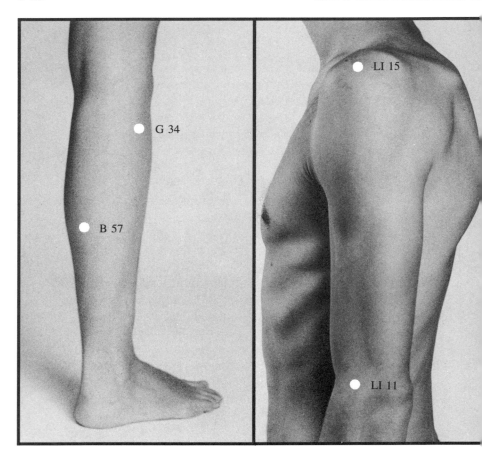

G 34 of the gall-bladder-meridian is called *Yang-lingquan*, "the Yang hill fountain"; it lies in the hollow between the calf and the shin-bone, two cun below the knee. *B 57* of the bladder-meridian is at the apex of an acute angle, a 'V' upside-down, that hollows out below the calf-muscle when you stretch your foot.

LI 15 of the large intestine-meridian lies between the outer end of the collar-bone and the bone of the arm, in a hollow that becomes apparent when the arm is raised. It can be acupressed for pain in both arm and shoulder. *LI 11* of the large intestine-meridian, called *Quchi*, "the pool at the bend," is at the outer end of the elbow flexor-fold and can be located by bending the arm.

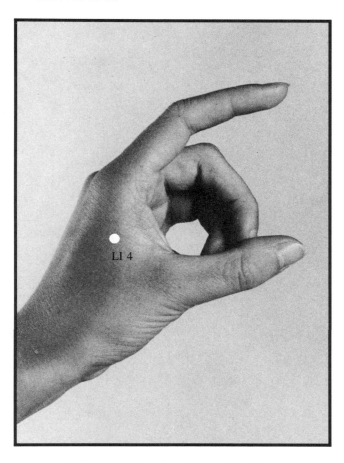

LI 4 of the large intestine meridian is located by putting your finger on the top of the hillock that appears when you press the thumb and fingers of the other hand against one another; you acupress after relaxing the hand. LI 4 is one of the oldest and most versatile acupoints; it is called *He*gu, ''the enclosed valley.'' Use it for arm and shoulder pains alike.

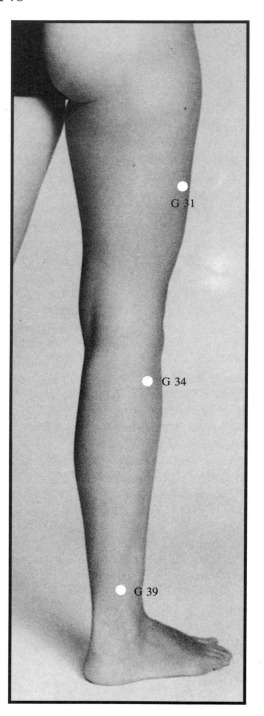

G 31 of the gall-bladder-meridian is the point you touch with your middle-finger if you let your arm hang at your side.
G 34 of the gall-bladder-meridian is at the front lower edge of the fibula-head.
G 39 of the gall-bladder-meridian, called *Kuanzhong*, "the swinging bell," lies three cun above the ankle-bone on the outer side behind the fibula.

G 30 of the gall-bladder-meridian is called *Huantiao*, "the leaping circle." It lies at the upper end of the neck of the femur. If you lie on your side, with the leg beneath you straight and the other bent, you can feel in the latter the thickening at the top of the femur, that of the greater trochanter. If you divide the distance from the coccyx to the trochanter by three, G 30 will be one-third away from the outer end of the line (illustration on opposite page)

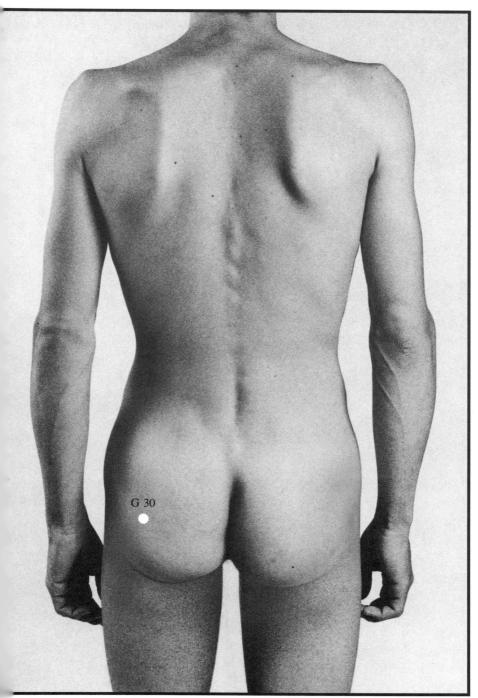

G 30

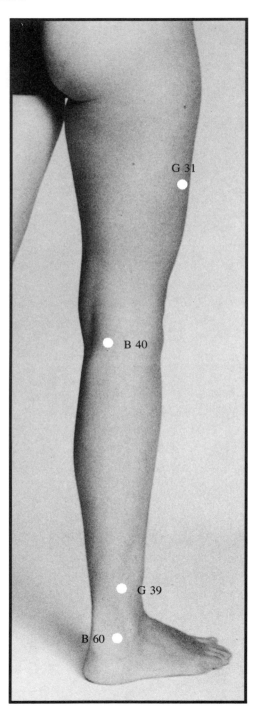

G 31 of the gall-bladder-meridian is the point you touch with your middle-finger if you stand straight and let your arms dangle at your sides. *B 40* of the bladder-meridian is in the center of the flexor-fold of the knee. *G 39* of the gall-bladder-meridian is behind the fibula, three cun above the ankle-bone. *B 60* of the bladder-meridian is called *Kunlun*, which is the name of a Chinese mountain; it is on the same level as the ankle-bone, just before the Achilles-tendon.

G 30 of the gall-bladder-meridian lies two-thirds of the distance from the coccyx to the greater trochanter, the upper thickening of the femur, on the edge of the neck of the femur. To locate the greater trochanter, lie on your side with the leg beneath you straight and the other bent (illustration on opposite page)

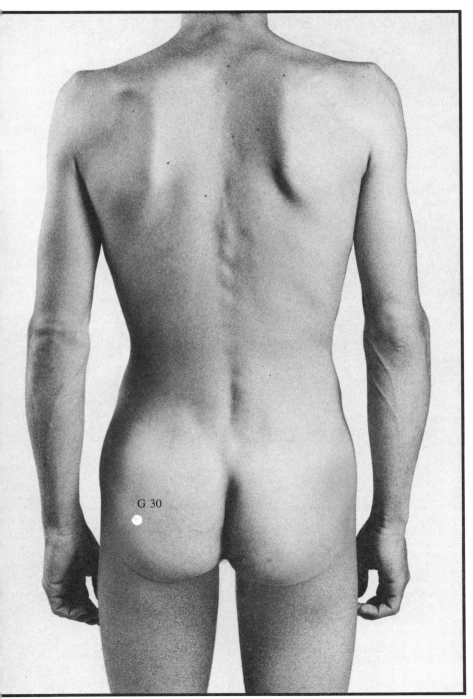

G 30

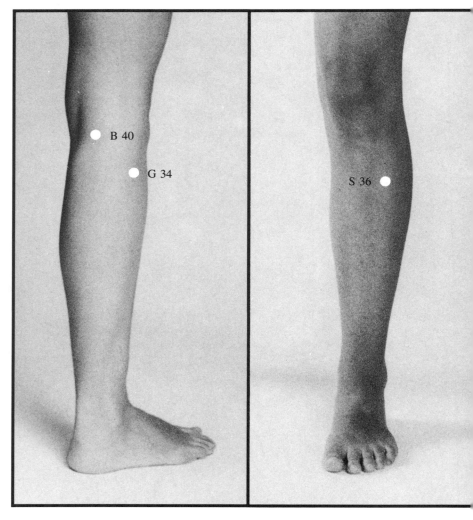

B 40 of the bladder-meridian is in the middle of the flexor-fold of the knee. *G 34* of the gall-bladder-meridian, called *Yanglingquan*, ''the Yang hill spring,'' lies in a hollow at the front lower edge of the head of the fibula.

S 36 of the stomach-meridian lies three cun down from the lower edge of the knee-cap then one cun outwards. It is much appreciated as a point of overall tonification and is utilised for therapy in many fields.

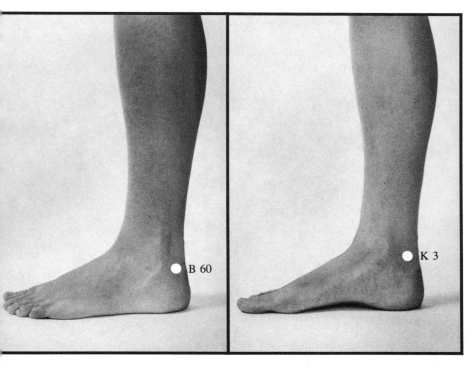

B 60 of the bladder-meridian, with the name of the mountain *Kunlun*, lies in the hollow between the outer end of the ankle-bone and the Achilles-tendon.

K 3 of the kidney-meridian lies between the ankle-bone and the Achilles-tendon on the inner side. Be careful to keep on the same level as the ankle-bone when locating it, otherwise you may acupress *K4* by mistake, only half a cun further down!

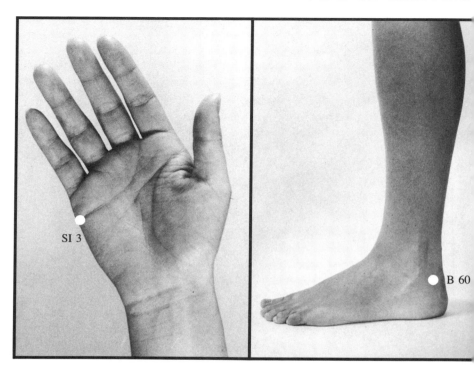

SI 3 of the small intestine-meridian is on the edge of the palm at the end of the uppermost transversal line. You can locate it immediately by closing your fist.

B 60 of the bladder-meridian is in the hollow between the ankle-bone and the Achilles-tendon on the outer side.

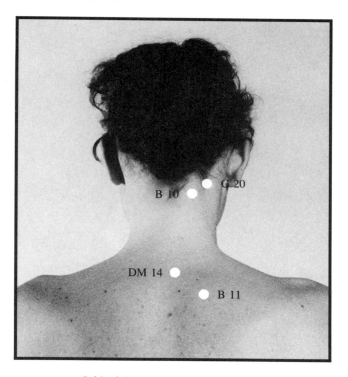

G 20 of the gall-bladder-meridian lies
in the hollow beside the trapeze-muscle
at the root of the hair. *B 10* of the
bladder-meridian is on the other side
of the same muscle, on an oblique lines
below *G 20. DM 14* of the Du Mai-
meridian is in the hollow below the
seventh cervical vertebra: *B 11* of the
bladder-meridian is a cun and a half
to the side of the following vertebra
and its spinous process.

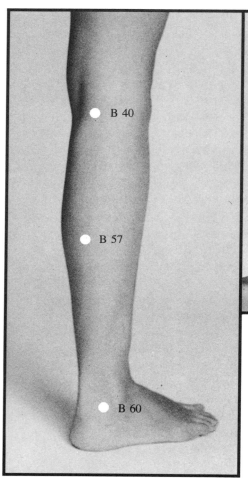

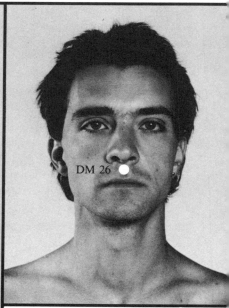

DM 26 of the Du Mai-meridian is two-thirds of the distance from the upper lip to the nose, in the center.

B 40 of the bladder-meridian is in the middle of the flexor-fold of the knee. B 57 of the bladder-meridian is at the apex of a triangular hollow that forms below the calf-muscle when you stretch your foot. B 60 of the bladder-meridian, the *Kunlun* acupoint, lies between the ankle-bone and the Achilles-tendon on the outer side.

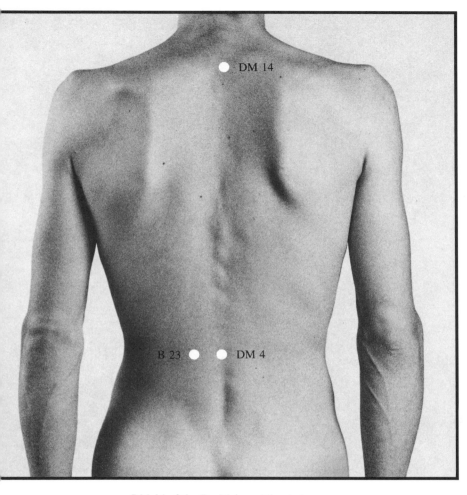

DM 14 of the Du Mai-meridian is in the hollow below the spinous process of the seventh cervical vertebra. *DM 4* of the Du Mai-meridian, called *Mingmen*, "the gate of life," lies between the spinous processes of the second and third lumbar vertebrae. *B 23* of the bladder-meridian is beside it, on the same level, a cun and a half further from the spine. The third lumbar vertebra in your back is on the same level as your navel in front.

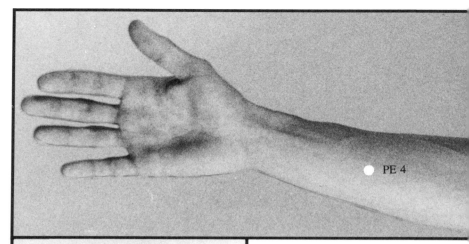

PE 4

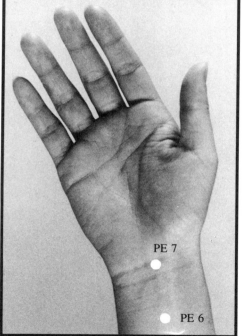

PE 7

PE 6

PE 4 of the pericardium-meridian lies five cun up the inner side of the forearm from the flexor fold at the wrist.

B 15 of the bladder-meridian is a cun and a half to the side of the fifth thoracic vertebra. It may be difficult to locate and acupress without the help of a second person and it will be easier for the latter if you bend your back so that the vertebrae stand out and can be counted. (Top, opposite page 159)

RM 17 of the Ren Mai-meridian is on the sternum in the center of the chest between the nipples. *RM 12* of the Ren Mai-meridian is half-way from the navel to the sternum. *LV 14* of the liver-meridian is in the hollow before the junction of sixth and seventh rib. It will be easiest to locate these three points when you are lying down. (Bottom, opposite page 159)

PE 6 of the pericardium-meridian, called *Neiguan,* "the inner link" is two cun up the arm from the flexor-fold and *PE 7* of the pericardium-meridian lies on the fold itself, in the center of the wrist. *PE 7* is called *Daling,* "the big hill."

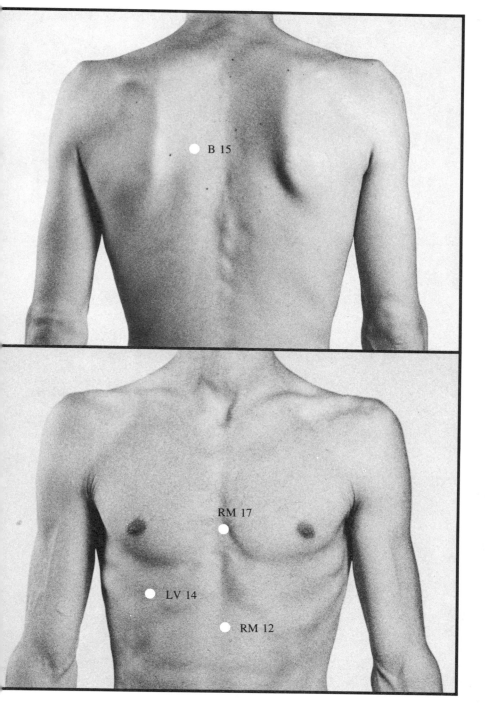

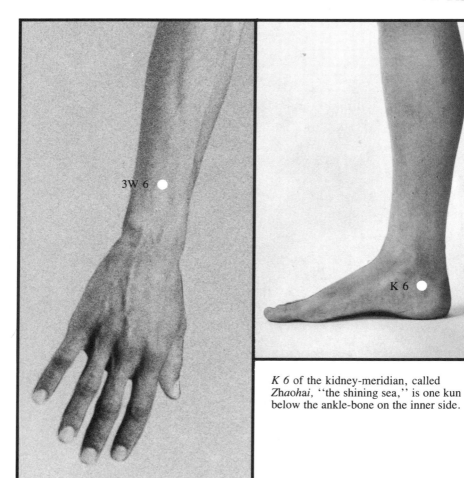

K 6 of the kidney-meridian, called Zhaohai, "the shining sea," is one kun below the ankle-bone on the inner side.

3W 6 of the tripartite warmer-meridian lies three cun from the wrist between ulna and radius on the outer side of the forearm. If you bend the arm as though you were carrying it in a sling the two bones will lie parallel and the hollow between them will be more marked than in any other position.

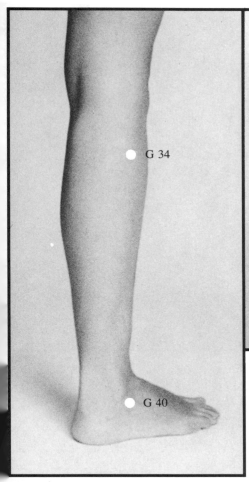

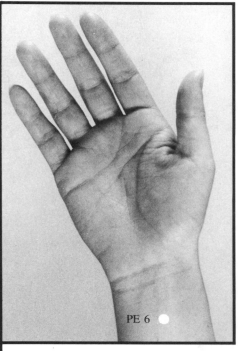

PE 6 of the pericardium-meridian, called *Neiguan*, "the inner link," is two cun above the center of the first flexor-fold of the wrist, on the inner side of the forearm.

G 34 of the gall-bladder-meridian lies at the lower edge of the head of the fibula in front. *G 40* of the gall-bladder-meridian, called *Qiuzu*, "the great wall," is in the hollow located obliquely below the ankle-bone on the outer side.

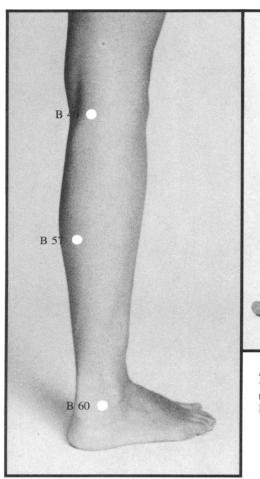

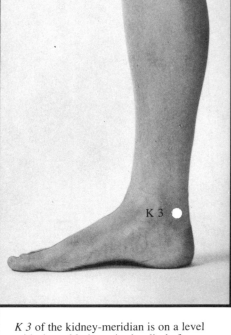

K 3 of the kidney-meridian is on a level with the ankle-bone in the dip before the Achilles-tendon on the inner side. It is called *Taixi*, ''the mighty stream.''

B 40 of the bladder-meridian lies behind the knee, in center of the flexor-fold. *B 57* of the bladder-meridian lies at the apex of a triangular hollow, a V upside-down, that forms below the calf-muscle when you stretch your foot. *B 60* of the bladder-meridian is in the dip between the ankle-bone and the Achilles-tendon on the outer side.

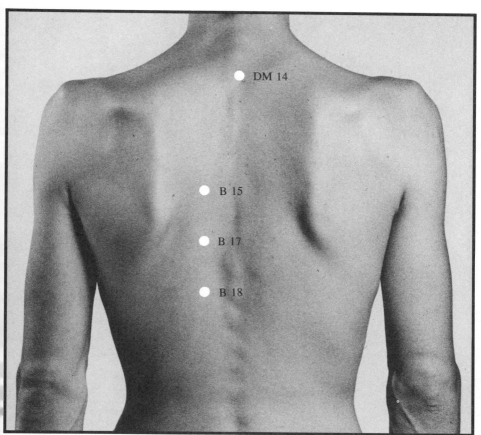

DM 14 of the Du Mai-meridian lies in the hollow between the seventh cervical vertebra and the first thoracic vertebra. *B15* of the bladder-meridian is beside the spinous process of the fifth thoracic vertebra, *B 17* beside that of the seventh and B 18 beside that of the ninth thoracic vertebra. These three points are all one cun and a half from the axial line. Bend your back to assist a partner in locating them.

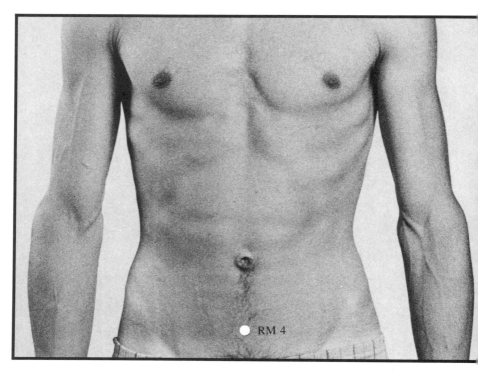

RM 4 of the Ren Mai-meridian is on
the axial line three cun below the navel.
It is called *Guanyuan*, ''the pivot of
life'' and is considered a tonification
point for the whole organism.

DIGESTION

We may think much of the physician's art, be it that of the East or of the West, and yet the medicine we administer to ourselves in our daily food is of infinitely greater value. Food that is lacking in variety or, as in Third-World countries, insufficient in quantity, throws open the gates to disease.

Even in the prosperous Western world, questions of nutrition and consequently of digestion leave much to be desired. Whereas Third-World poverty can lead to famine, abundance and almost unlimited consumer-facilities can lead to health problems due to over-eating and incorrect diet; quality is far from being in line with quantity. We eat too much sugar, fat, salt, protein, and not enough ballast to cleanse and activate the intestine. Many disorders of the digestive tract and the cardiovascular system can be avoided by a balanced diet and as much variety as possible. There can be no energy balance until the two factors of 'too much' or 'too little' have been eliminated. Basically, the Chinese concept of a balanced diet is in line with the thought expressed by Paracelsus, the XVIth. century physician, when he wrote:"In all things there is a poison, and there is no thing where poison is not. It depends entirely on the amount of the dose for a poison to be poisonous or not."

For us, the life-forces have three components: genetic energy, inherited from our parents, cosmic energy, received from the atmosphere, and nutritive energy, received from the food we eat. Good digestion depends not only on the quality of the food, but also on our frame of mind. So you should never think about your work while you are eating, and not before you have had at least a pause to digest your food afterwards.

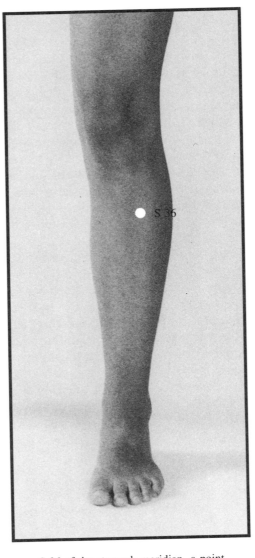

S 36 of the stomach-meridian, a point
of overall tonification, lies three cun
below the lower edge of the knee-cap
and then one cun to the outer side.

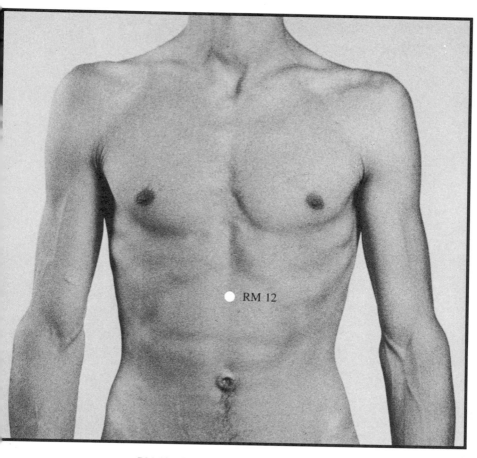

RM 12 of the Ren Mai-meridian is on
the axial line between the edge of the
sternum and the navel. It is called
Zhongwan, "the stomach's center."

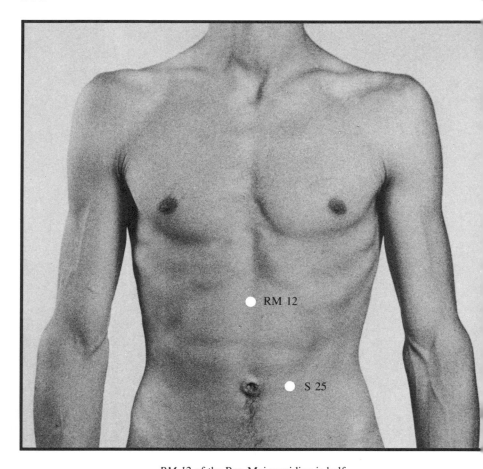

RM 12 of the Ren Mai-meridian is half-
way between the edge of the sternum
and the navel. It is easiest to locate when
lying down so that the trunk is stretched
out. *S 25* of the stomach-meridian,
called *Tianshu,* ''the axis of heaven,''
lies two cun to the side of the navel,
on the same level.

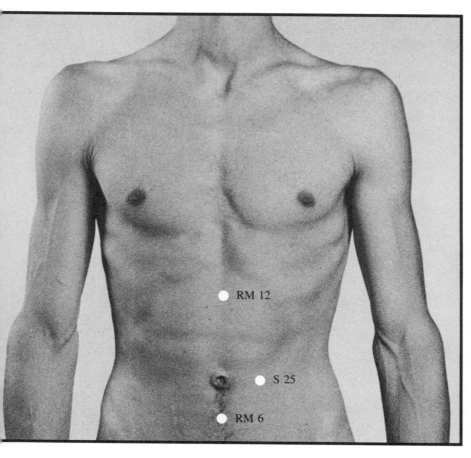

RM 12 of the Ren Mai-meridian, called
Zhongwan, is half-way between the
edge of the sternum and the navel, on
the axial line. *S 25* of the stomach-
meridian, *Tianshu,* is two cun to the
side of the navel, on the same level.
RM 6 of the Ren Mai-meridian, called
Qihai, ''the sea of energy,'' is a cun
and a half below the navel. All these
points should be located lying down so
that the body is stretched out.

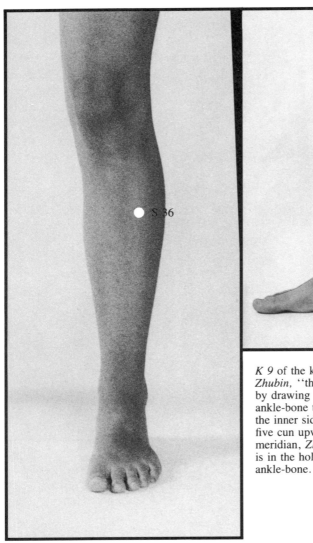

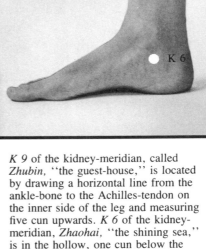

K 9 of the kidney-meridian, called *Zhubin*, "the guest-house," is located by drawing a horizontal line from the ankle-bone to the Achilles-tendon on the inner side of the leg and measuring five cun upwards. K 6 of the kidney-meridian, *Zhaohai*, "the shining sea," is in the hollow, one cun below the ankle-bone.

S 36 of the stomach-meridian is the point of overall tonification that lies three cun below the knee and then one cun outwards on the same level.

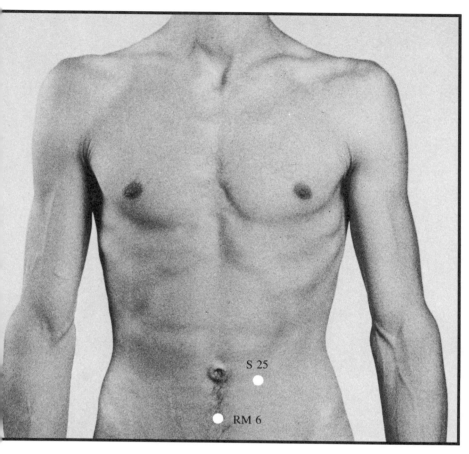

S 25

RM 6

S 25 of the stomach-meridian, called
Tianshu, "the axis of heaven," is on
a line with the navel, two cun away.
RM 6 of the Ren Mai-meridian, called
Qihai, "the sea of energy," lies a cun
and a half below the navel.

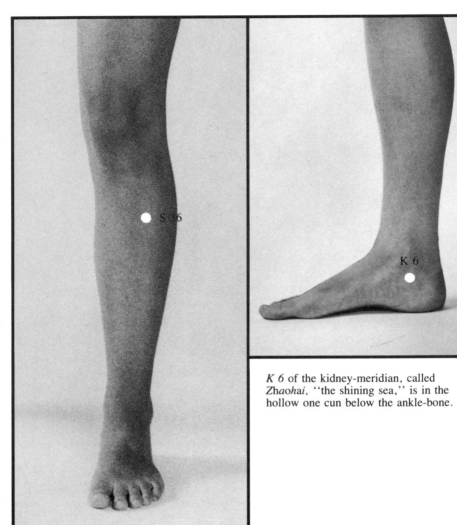

K 6 of the kidney-meridian, called
Zh*aohai*, "the shining sea," is in the
hollow one cun below the ankle-bone.

S 36 of the stomach-meridian is located
three cun down from the knee-cap and
then one cun outwards.

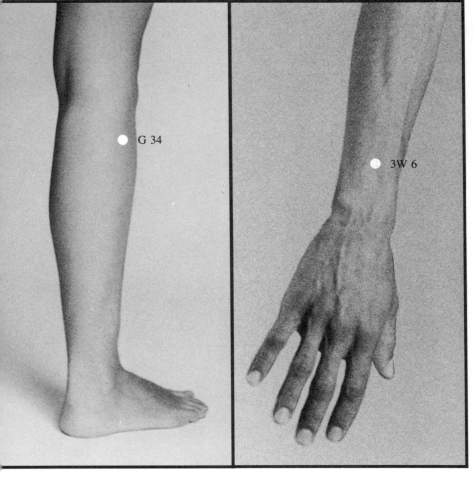

G 34 of the gall-bladder-meridian, called *Yanglingquan*, "the Yang hill spring," is in a hollow below the front edge of the head of the fibula.

3W 6 of the tripartite-warmer, which is a Yang-meridian of the hand, lies three cun from the wrist on the outer side of the arm in the hollow between ulna and radius; to locate it, these two bones must be parallel, with the arm bent as though lying in a sling.

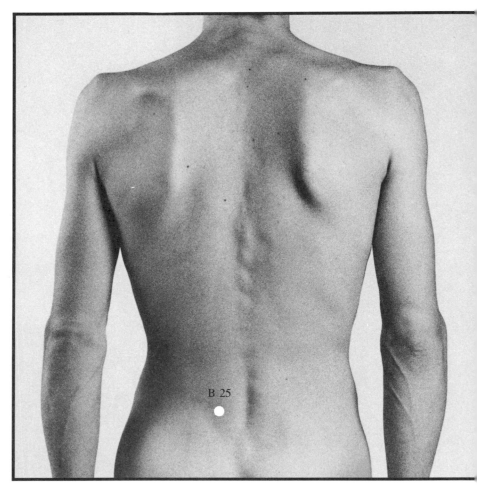

B 25 of the bladder-meridian lies a cun
and a half away from the spinous process
of the fourth lumbar vertebra, on a level
with the top of the pelvic bone.

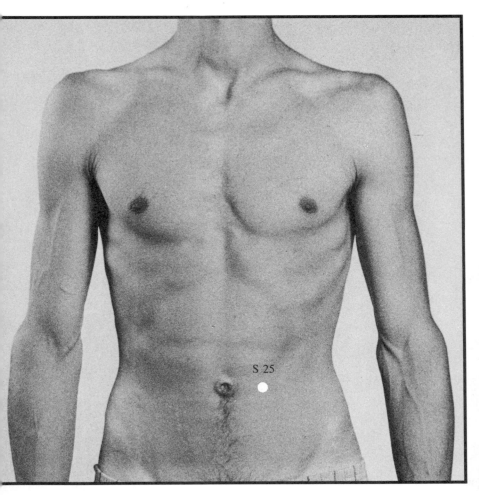

S 25 of the stomach-meridian, "the heavenly axis," is on a level with the navel, two cun to the side.

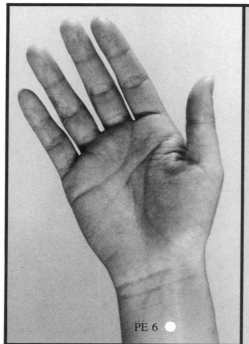

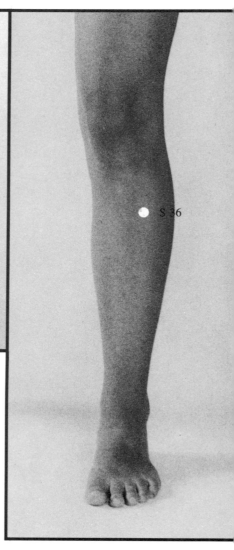

PE 6 of the pericardium-meridian is in the middle of the forearm on the inner side, two cun from the first flexor-fold of the wrist.

S 36 of the stomach-meridian lies three cun below the knee-cap and one cun to the side of that point.

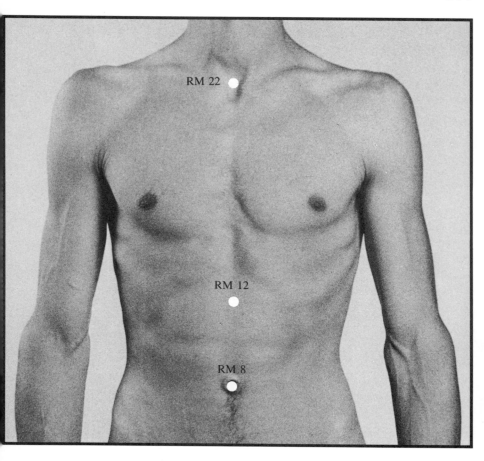

RM 22 of the Ren Mai-meridian is half a cun above the top of the sternum at the throat. *RM 12* lies on the axial line midway between the sternum and the navel. *RM 8*, called "the palace of the spirit," *Shenque*, is in the navel; direct pressure on the point, where acupuncture is prohibited, must be avoided; massage round it with the palm of the hand.

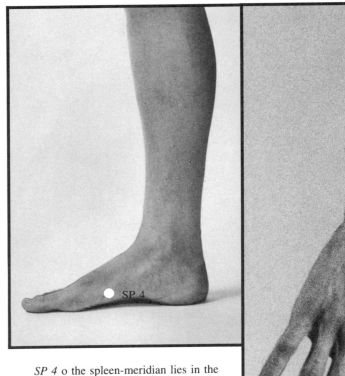

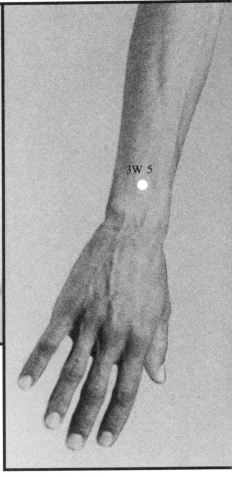

SP 4 o the spleen-meridian lies in the hollow at the root of the metatarsal bone of the big toe, on the color-line between the darker, well irrigated sole of the foot and the upper part.

3W 5 of the tripartite warmer, which is called *Waiguan,* "the outer link," lies between ulna and radius two cun above the wrist on the outer side of the forearm.

THE RESPIRATORY TRACT

Our food and the work of the digestive system provide us with energy from the earth; the respiratory system links us with the universe, we are receiving cosmic forces together with the air we breathe. We have a built-in filtering-plant, which is our nose, to protect us from wind and weather. The nose monitors the air-temperature as we breathe it and keeps dust and germs away from our pharynx and throat. Consequently, it is usually the place where we catch a cold. Even then, we must make every effort to go on breathing through the nose and to prevent it at all costs from becoming completely blocked. Once we start breathing through the mouth all the painful symptoms of the cold will break out in full force.

Timely acupressure to free the respiratory tract is preventive and curative at the same time. It rids us of the unpleasant symptom of swollen mucous and protects the pharynx and throat from renewed infection as well as from the effects of the cold, windy, or dry atmosphere. The old Chinese proverb says: "Keep out of the way of the wind and the flying arrow" and I need hardly remind you how slight a draught can be the cause of a sore throat.

Some people have a nose that is constantly stuffed up, even when they do not have a cold; they may indeed be unaware of the fact. It may be due to chronic sinusitis of varying degrees of gravity. The sufferers concerned frequently complain that their sense of smell is impaired and they often have a heavy head and feel oppressed. Acupressure is particularly effective in these cases; usually the nose begins to run while the first acupoints are being massaged; the air-passage is free and there is no more pressure in the head.

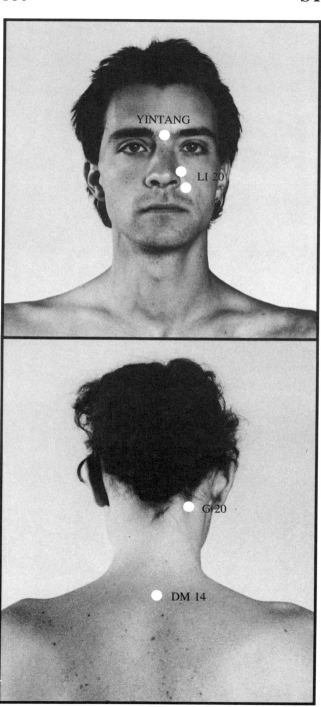

Yintang is in the center between the eyebrows; it is a special point, unconnected with any meridian. The upper and lower *LI 20* of the large intestine-meridian lie, one above the nostril, one below it, on the oblique line running from the nose to the corner of the mouth.

G 20 of the gall-bladder-meridian is in the hollow on the outer side of the trapeze-muscle. Move your head from side to side to locate it. *DM 14* of the Du Mai-meridian is in the hollow below the seventh cervical vertebra, the one that is prominent when you bend your head.

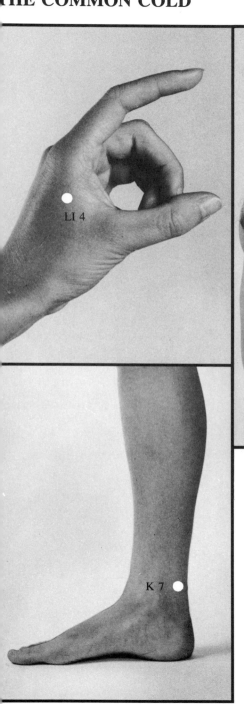

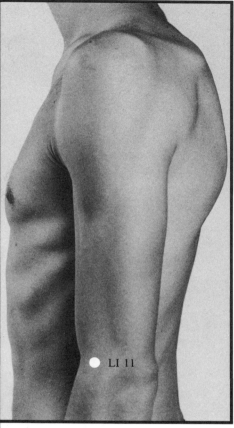

LI 4 of the large intestine-meridian, on the metacarpus-bone of the forefinger is acupressed both for nose-blockage and for a cold in the head.

K 7 of the kidney-meridian, called *Fuliu,* "the returning stream," is located by taking a horizontal line from the ankle-bone to the Achilles-tendon and measuring two cun up vertically in the hollow.

LI 11 of the large intestine-meridian, called *Quchi,* "the pool at the bend," is located with your arm bent and lies between the outer end of the flexor-fold and the head of the humerus.

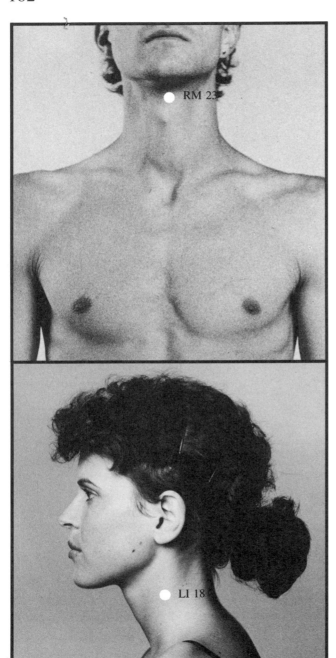

RM 23 of the Ren Mai-meridian is on the throat, half-way between the top of the Adam's apple and the lower edge of the maxillary.

LI 18 of the large-intestine-meridian is on a level with the Adam's apple, three cun back round the throat.

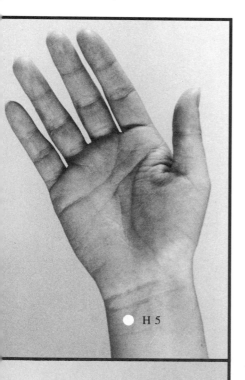

H 5 of the heart-meridian, called *Tongl*i, ''inner understanding,'' is on the outer side of the ligament connecting the ulna with the wrist, one cun beyond the flexor-fold.

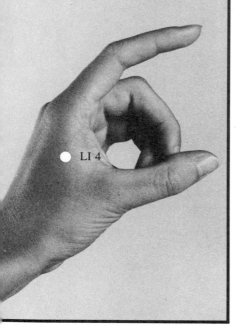

LI 4 of the large intestine-meridian is on the metacarpus of the forefinger, at the point standing out when you press the thumb against the hand. Acupress with the forefinger of the other hand.

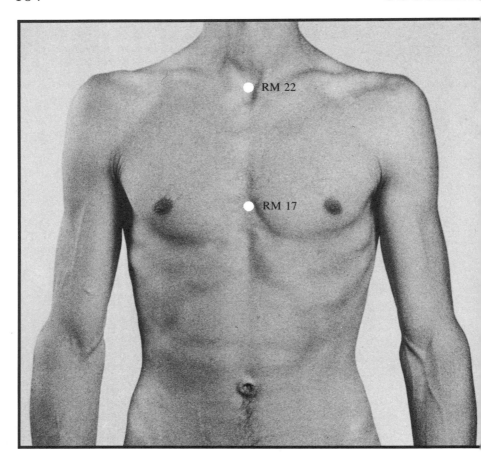

RM 22 of the Ren Mai-meridian is in
the jugular fossa, half a cun above the
sternum. *RM 17* of the Ren Mai meridian
is on the axial line between the nipples
and is best located when lying down.

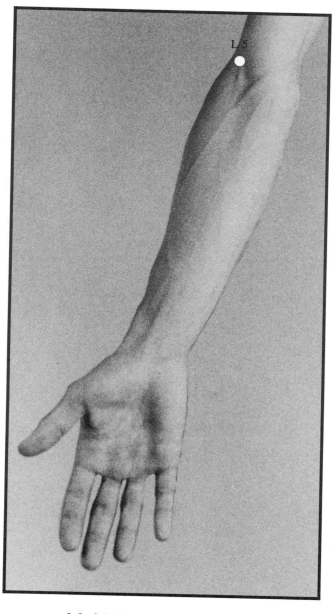

L 5 of the lung-meridian is located
beside the biceps in the elbow flexor-
fold. Bend the arm slightly and it will
be easy to find.

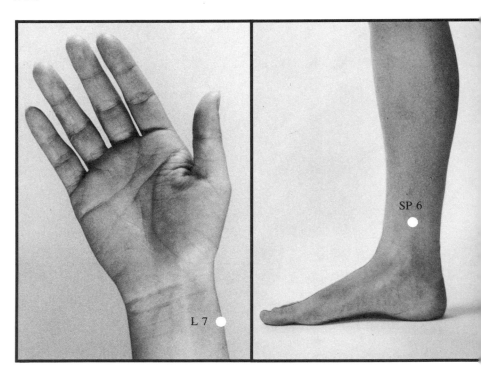

L 7 of the lung-meridian lies a cun and a half above the wrist flexor-fold in a hollow at the upper edge of the radius articulation. You touch the point with your forefinger when you cross your hands thumb to thumb.

SP 6 of the spleen-meridian is behind the shinbone on the inner side of the leg, three cun above the ankle-bone.

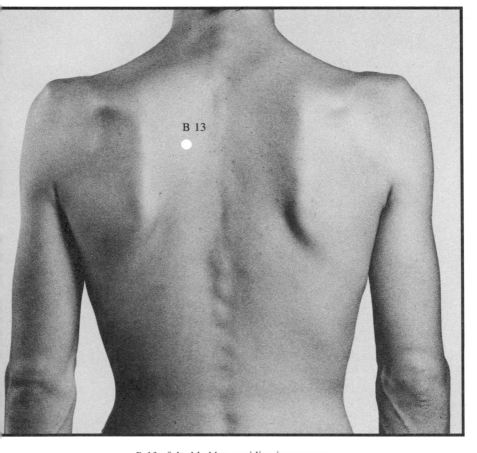

B 13 of the bladder-meridian is one cun and a half to the side of the spinous process of the third thoracic vertebra. If you need the help of a second person to locate and acupress this point, it is best to bend your back and head so that the vertebrae stand out; the seventh cervical is the most prominent and the thoracic vertebrae start immediately below it.

UROGENITAL DISORDERS

The urogenital system, as we see things in China, lies wholly in the operational area of the kidneys. When the kidneys are weakened, people are prone to diseases of the bladder and the urinary tract, but there may likewise be a tendency to sexual debility and complaints of the genitalia. The urogenital organs are highly sensitive in every respect and they are often the first to react to psychic problems: in times of stress, some women find that their monthly cycle is completely out of tune; impotence in men is frequently a case for the psycho-analyst rather than the physician; a state of fear can cause enuresis in adults as well as in children.

The reverse situation also applies: the mind reacts with extreme sensitivity to any ailment of the urogenital system. Urgency of micturation, due to cystitis or disorders of the prostrate, distresses people so much that they will not even speak of it. Hormonal changes at the time of the climacteric can lead to serious psychic troubles in women; painful or excessive menstruation-flow may cause depression. Most suf-ferers from sexual complaints refuse to discuss their troubles except in writing; the letters the sex-counsellors answer through the media are doubtless signed with an imaginary name but they describe very real ailments.

In acupressure-therapy for urogenital complaints, I combine in the first place the meridians directly concerned, those of the bladder and the kidneys, with adjacent points on the Ren Mai-meridian, where perturbations of the energy-flow may also produce symptoms in the urogenital field. In addition I use points of overall tonification, such as *S 36* of the stomach-meridian and some distant points of other meridians.

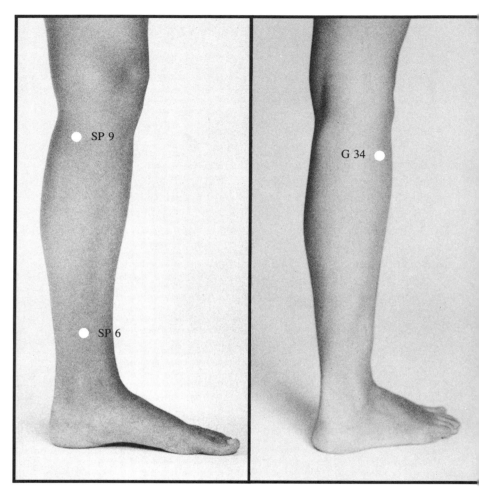

SP 9 of the spleen-meridian, called *Yinlingquan,* ''the Yin hill spring,'' is in a hollow behind the head of the shinbone, which you can feel beside the knee on the inner side. *SP 6* of the spleen-meridian lies exactly three cun above the ankle-bone, behind the shinbone, on the inner side of the leg.

G 34 of the gall-bladder-meridian, called *Yanglingquan,* ''the Yang hill spring,'' is at the front lower edge of the head of the fibula.

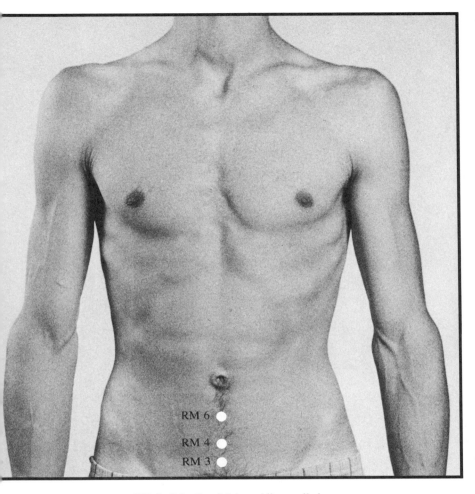

RM 6
RM 4
RM 3

RM 6 of the Ren Mai meridian, called *Qihai*, "the sea of energy," is a cun and a half below the navel.

RM 4 is three cun below the navel and is called *Guanyuan*, "the pivot of life." *RM 3*, called *Zhangji*, "the extreme center," lies one cun further down. These three Ren Mai points are easiest to locate when lying down.

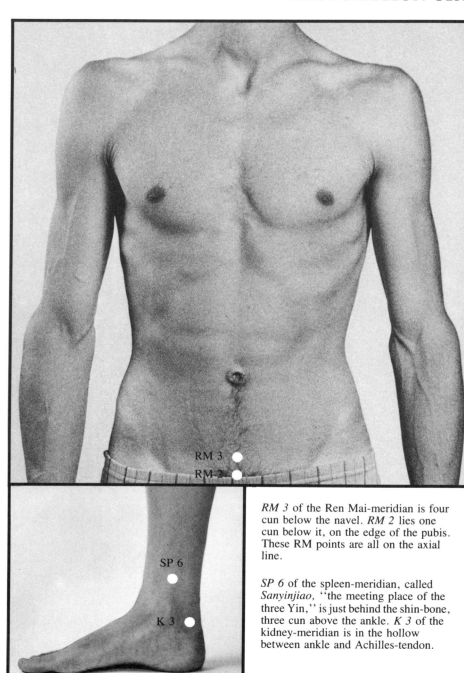

RM 3 of the Ren Mai-meridian is four cun below the navel. *RM 2* lies one cun below it, on the edge of the pubis. These RM points are all on the axial line.

SP 6 of the spleen-meridian, called *Sanyinjiao*, ''the meeting place of the three Yin,'' is just behind the shin-bone, three cun above the ankle. *K 3* of the kidney-meridian is in the hollow between ankle and Achilles-tendon.

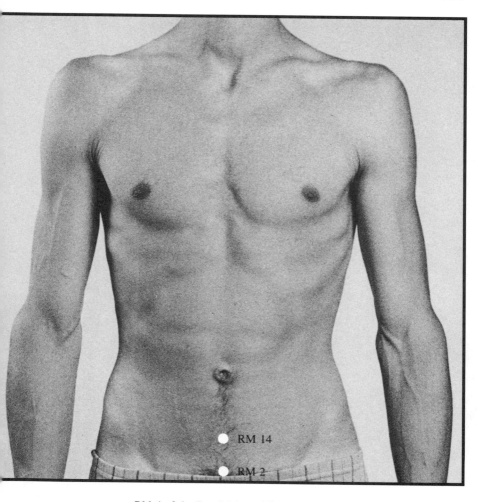

RM 14

RM 2

RM 4 of the Ren Mai-meridian, called
"the pivot of life," *Guanyuan,* is three
cun below the navel; *RM 2,* called *Qugu,*
"the crooked bone," is five cun below
the navel, on the edge of the pubis.
These axial-line points are best located
when lying down.

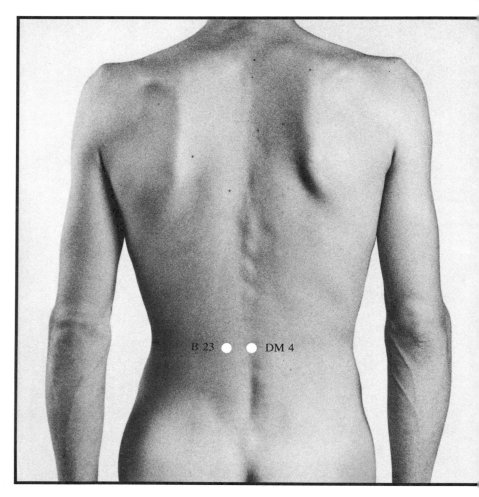

DM 4 of the Du Mai-meridian, called *Mingmen,* "the gate of life," lies between the spinous process of the second lumbar vertebra and that of the third. *B 23* of the bladder-meridian is a cun and a half to the side of the second lumbar vertebra spinous process.

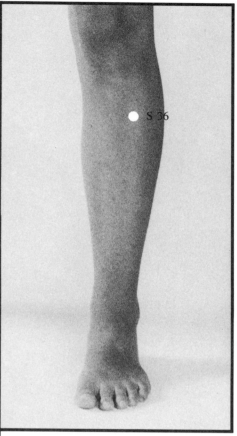

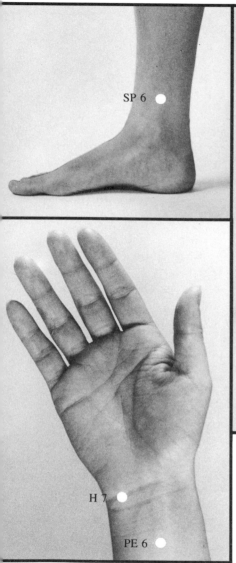

SP 6 of the spleen-meridian lies behind the shin-bone, three cun above the ankle-bone. SP 6 is the point where the spleen-meridian meets the two other Yin-meridians of the foot; it is called *Sanyinjiao*, "three Yin meeting-place" S 36 of the stomach-meridian is three cun below the knee-cap and one cun outwards from that point.

H 7 of the heart-meridian is on the outer side of the ligament connecting ulna and wrist, in the continuation of a line running from between the ring-finger and the little finger. *PE 6* of the pericardium-meridian is in the center of the forearm on the inner side, two cun from the first flexor-fold of the wrist.

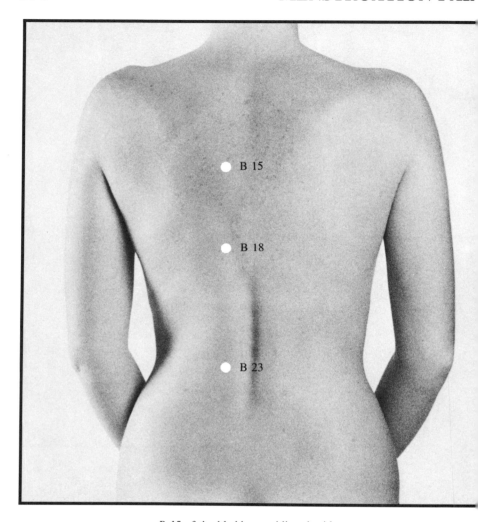

B 15 of the bladder-meridian, beside
the spinous process of the fifth thoracic
vertebra, *B 18* beside that of the ninth
thoracic vertebra, and *B 23* beside that
of the second lumbar vertebra, all lie
one cun and a half from the spinal axial
line.

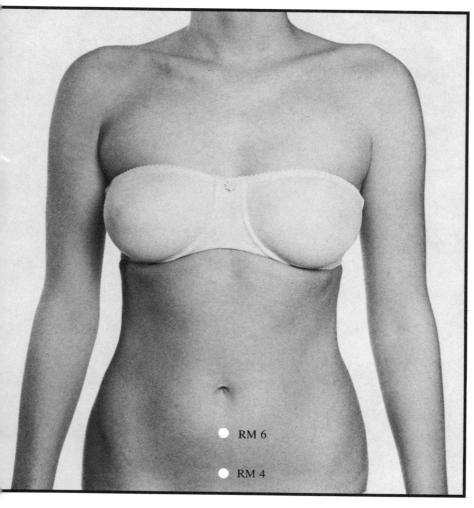

RM 6 of the Ren Mai-meridian, called *Qihai*, "the sea of energy," is one cun and a half below the navel; *RM 4*, *Guanyuan*, "the pivot of life" is three cun below the navel. Both are on the abdominal axial line.

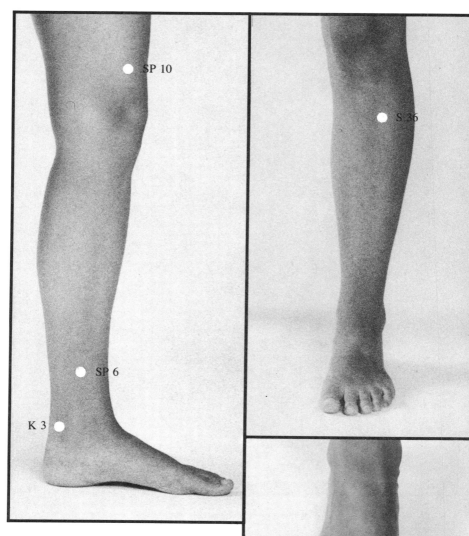

SP 10 of the spleen-meridian, called Xuehai, "the sea of blood," is two cun above the edge of the knee-cap on the inner side on the summit of the femur muscle. SP 6 of the spleen meridian, called Sanyinjiao, "the meeting-place of the three Yin," is three cun above the ankle behind the shin-bone. K 3 of the kidney-meridian is between the Achilles-tendon and the ankle-bone, on a level with the latter.

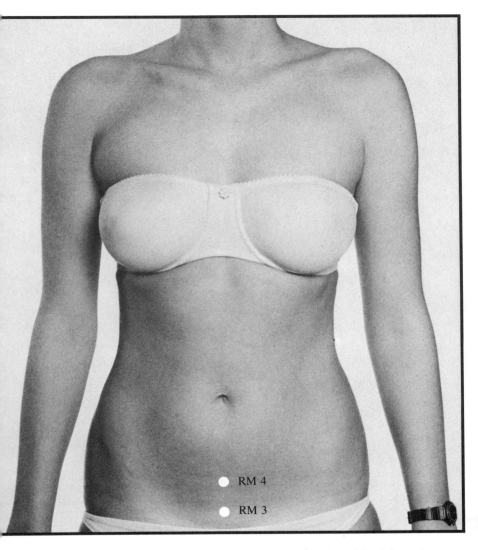

S 36 of the stomach-meridian is three cun below the knee-cap and one cun outwards from there. It is a much-appreciated point of overall tonification.

S 44 of the stomach-meridian lies half a cun from the space between the second and third toe. It is called *Neiting*, "the inner court."

RM 4 of the Ren Mai-meridian is located three cun below the navel; it is called *Guanyuan*, "the pivot of life." RM 3 of the Ren Mai-meridian, called *Zhongji*, "the extreme center," is four cun below the navel. Both points should be measured when lying down, so that the navel will be in its anatomically correct position and the abdomen flat.

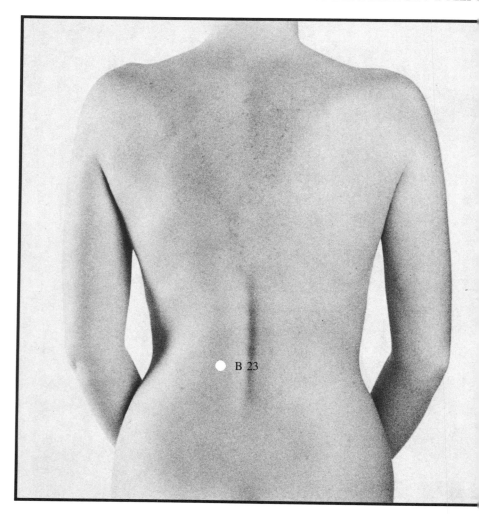

B 23 of the bladder-meridian lies one
cun and a half from from the spinous
process of the second lumbar vertebra
on the same level, which corresponds
to that of the navel on the other side
of your body.

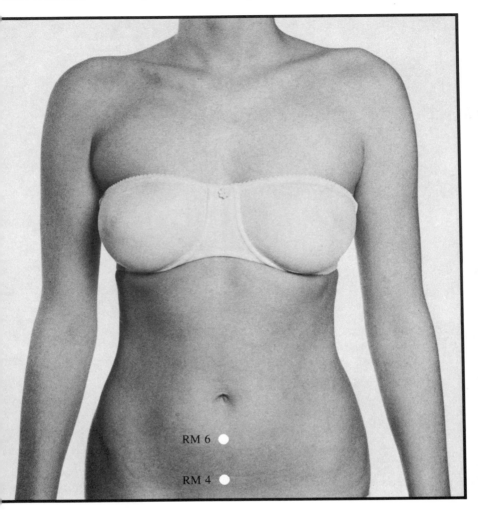

RM 6

RM 4

RM 6 of the Ren Mai-meridian lies a cun and a half below the navel; *RM 4* is three cun below the navel. Both points are on the abdominal axial line.

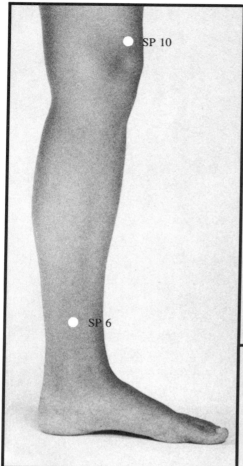

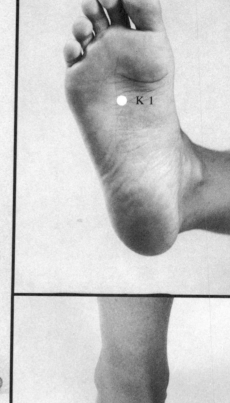

SP 10 of the spleen-meridian, called *Xuehai*, "the sea of blood," is two cun above the edge of the knee-cap on the inner side of the summit of the femur muscle. SP 6 is three cun above the ankle-bone, behind the shin-bone.

K 1, the starting-point of the kidney-meridian, is called *Yongquan*, "the gushing spring"; it lies in the center of the sole of the foot, two-thirds of the distance from the heel.

LV 1 of the liver-meridian and SP 1 of the spleen-meridian lie at the root of the big toe-nail, LV 1 at the inner side and SP 1 at the outer side

SKIN DISEASES

I wonder whether there is any sector of the Western economy that can boast quite as many similar and even identical products with as many different and more or less fanciful names as the Cosmetics industry. I could hardly believe my eyes when I first arrived in Europe and saw all these dermatologically and clinically tested, anti-allergic beauty-products, not to mention the accompanying publicity! These creams and lotions for "sensitive," or "delicate," or "damaged" skin, were "relaxing," or "stimulating" and they could "regenerate the tissues" and "curb the ageing process of the skin."

As we see things in China, a fine, healthy skin does not depend on the external application of preparations, but on nutrition, the air we breathe and the condition of our lungs. The lungs are regarded as the monitor of the skin and an unhealthy skin often indicates a functional debility of the lungs. The skin is always treated internally, both for prevention and as therapy for eczema, psoriasis and various other morbid conditions.

If any of the acupoints I shall be discussing in this chapter happen to be located at the focus of your particular trouble, be careful not to massage it but the corresponding point on the other half of your anatomy. I am also indicating here two sequences of acupoints which have proved effective for the treatment of eczema.

First series: Du Mai-meridian 14, large intestine-meridian 11, tripartite warmer-meridian 8, spleen-meridian 10, stomach-meridian 36.

Second series: Du Mai-meridian 20, large intestine-meridian 4, spleen-meridian 6, bladder-meridian 12, 13, and 40.

As therapy for psoriasis, begin by acupressing the eczema points and then the set of large intestine-meridian 4, liver-meridian 3 and heart-meridian 7.

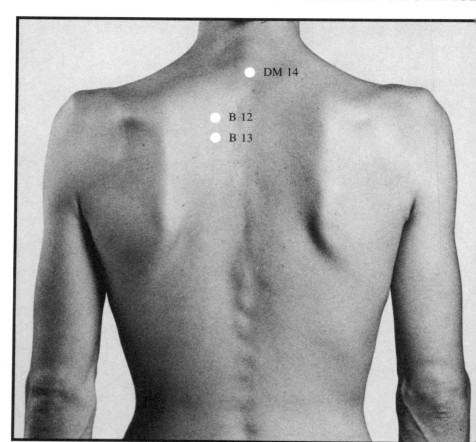

DM 14 of the Du Mai-meridian is just
below the spinous process of the seventh
cervical vertebra, the one that protrudes
when you bow your head; the point is
called *Dazhui,* ''big vertebra.'' *B12* and
B 13 of the bladder-meridian both lie
a cun and a half from the axial line, *B
12* beside the spinous process of the
second thoracic vertebra, *B 13* beside
that of the third thoracic vertebra.

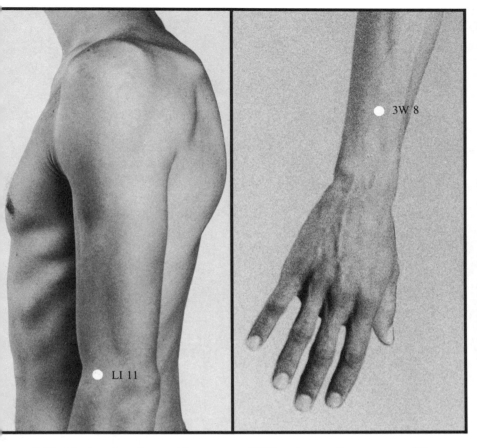

LI 11 of the large intestine-meridian can be felt when you bend your arm, at the inner end of the elbow flexor-fold.

3W 8 of the tripartite warmer-meridian is in the hollow between ulna and radius, four cun away from the wrist-fold on the outer side of the forearm. To locate it, bend the arm as though in a sling.

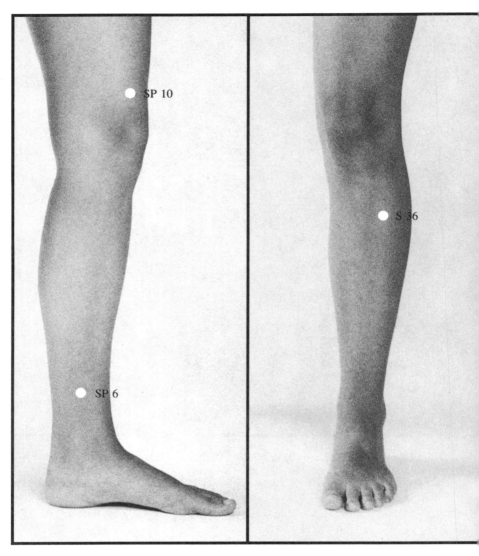

SP 10 of the spleen-meridian is on the summit of the thigh-bone muscle, two cun above the edge of the knee-cap on the inner side. SP 6 of the spleen-meridian is three cun above the ankle-bone behind the shin-bone.

S 36 of the stomach-meridian is three cun below the edge of the knee-cap and then one cun outwards.

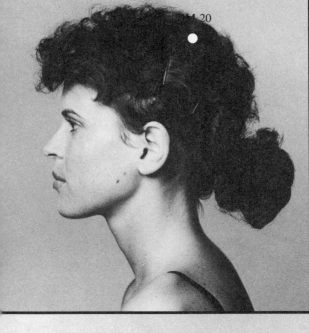

DM 20 of the Du Mai-
meridian, called Baíhuí,
''the point of one hundred
concordances,'' is located
by measuring eight cun
from the central point
between the eyebrows over
the forehead and the
vertex.

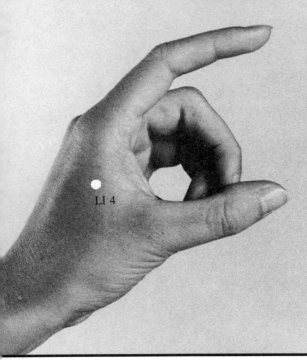

LI 4 of the large intestine
meridian is called Hegu,
''the enclosed valley''; it
lies on the metacarpus of
the forefinger and will be
on the summit of a hillock
formed by pressing the
thumb against the side of
the hand. Relax before
acupressing.

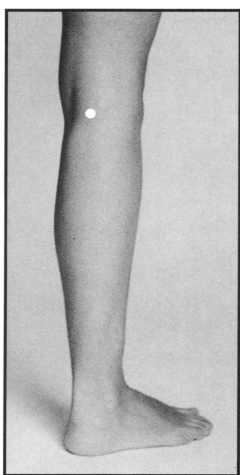

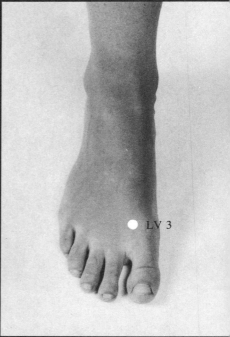

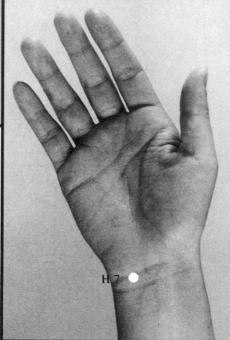

B 40 of the bladder-meridian is called *Weizhong*, "the hollow of the knee," and this is where it lies, in the center of the knee flexor-fold.

LV 3 of the liver-meridian, called *Taichong*, "flood-tide," is two cun away from the space between the big toe and the second toe.

H 7 of the heart-meridian is called *Shenmen*, "the gate of the spirit," It lies in the first flexor-fold of the wrist, on the outer side of the ligament connecting wrist and ulna.

VARICOSE VEINS

If the veins slacken, they cannot perform their function of returning used blood to the cells satisfactorily. There will be local congestion in the places where the walls of the veins are least elastic. The blood can coagulate, forming clots or plugs, there may be embolism or thrombosis threatening life itself. The condition is most dangerous when it is not discovered and given immediate treatment. Few people actually become seriously ill as the result of their varicose veins, but the thickening of the vessels is unesthetic and the side-effects, such as heavy, aching legs, are unpleasant. So we have every reason to do all we can to prevent them. Prevention is indeed the best advice that I can offer; anyone who already has varicose veins will find it well-nigh impossible to get rid of them.

Acupressure cannot heal them either, but it can relieve the accompanying symptoms and prevent them from growing worse. It must be practised daily if it is to be effective.

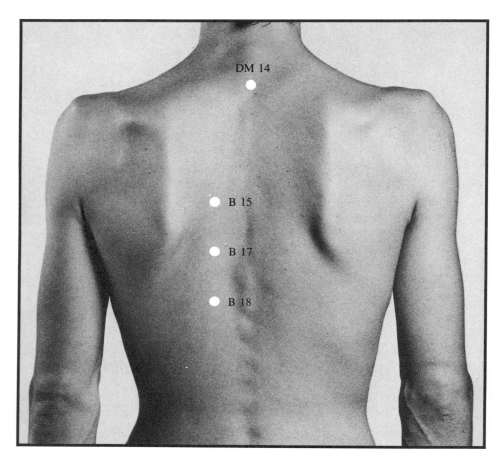

DM 14 of the Du Mai-meridian lies
below the spinous process of the seventh
cervical vertebra. *B 15, B 17, B 18* of
the bladder-meridian are all located a
cun and a half from the axial line, *B
15* on the level of the fifth thoracic
vertebra, *B 17* on that of the seventh,
B 18 on that of the ninth. Acupress with
the help of a second person; bend the
back to facilitate locating points.

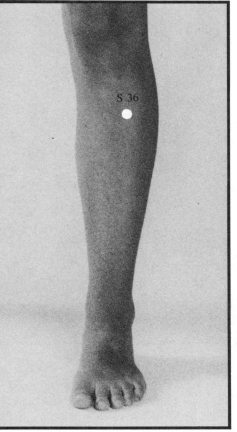

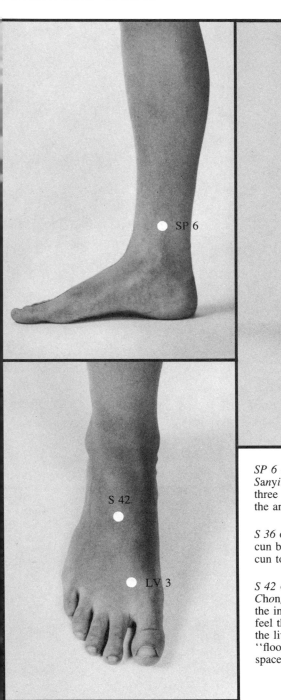

SP 6 of the spleen-meridian, called *Sanyinjiao*, "the meeting-point of the three Yin," is located three cun above the ankle-bone, on the inner side.

S 36 of the stomach-meridian lies three cun below the knee-cap and then one cun towards the outer side of the leg.

S 42 of the stomach-meridian, called *Chongyang*, "the rushing Yang," is on the instep at the point where you can feel the pulse of the artery. *LV 3* of the liver-meridian, called *Taichong*, "flood-tide," is two cun away from the space between the first and second toe.

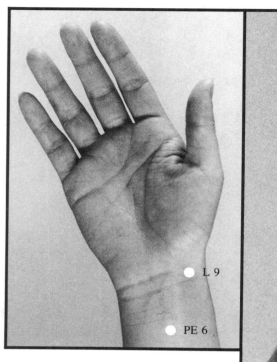

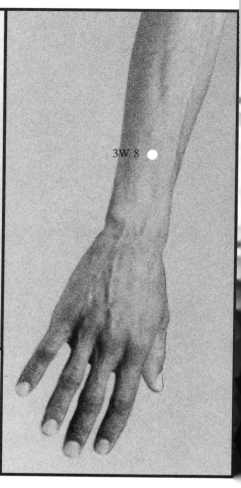

L 9 of the lung-meridian is called *Taiyuan*, ''the deepest chasm''; it lies in the hollow that can be felt at the wrist-fold beside the pulse of the radius, when the hand is bent back. *Pe 6* of the pericardium-meridian lies in the center of the forearm, on the inner side, two cun above the first flexor-fold of the wrist.

3W 8 of the tripartite warmer-meridian lies four cun above the wrist on the outer side of the arm, between ulna and radius in a hollow that is easiest to locate when the arm is bent as though carried in a sling.

INFLAMMATION OF THE EYES

To be correct, we should speak of inflammation of the conjunctiva, the membrane lining the eyelid and covering the eyeball; inflammation of the eye itself required immediate medical treatment. An iritis, an internal infection of the eye, can lead to cataract or glaucoma unless it is given treatment straight away. An inflammation of the cornea is apt to leave permanent scars that affect the eyesight. These complaints are usually so painful in any case that the sufferer will need no persuasion to visit his doctor, as I am sure anyone who has had snow-blindness will readily confirm.

When people speak of inflammation of the eye, they usually are not referring to disorders of the eyeball but to an itching, irritating swelling and redness of the eyelids and the conjunctiva. The causes are manifold. A speck of dust can irritate our eyes to such an extent that we keep rubbing them and produce acute inflammation. The air in some restaurants or bars may be so thick with smoke that people with sensitive eyes have to leave. Conjunctivitis may be due to bacteria or to a virus.

An allergic conjunctivitis may likewise be of a seasonal nature, caused by pollen in early summer. Carelessness in applying or removing eye-shadow and mascara may lead to chronic inflammation. Dirty hands are a permanent hazard. This is particularly important to remember when you acupress points anywhere near the eyes. Always wash your hands first and keep your nails fairly short.

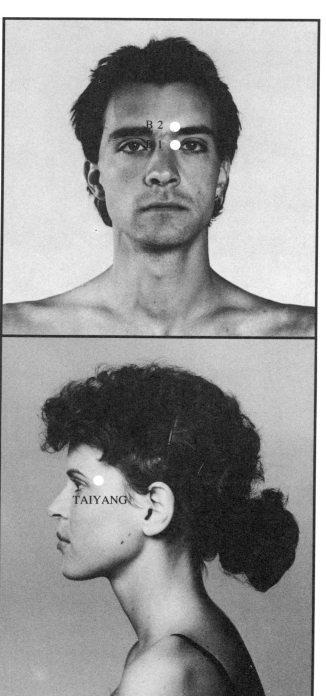

B 1 of the bladder-meridian is in the corner of the eye beside the nose *B 2* of the bladder-meridian is immediately above it in a hollow at th end of the eyebrow.

Taiyang is a special point, outside the meridian-system. It lies between the outer corner of the eye and the eyebrow, in the hollow behind the zygomatic bone.

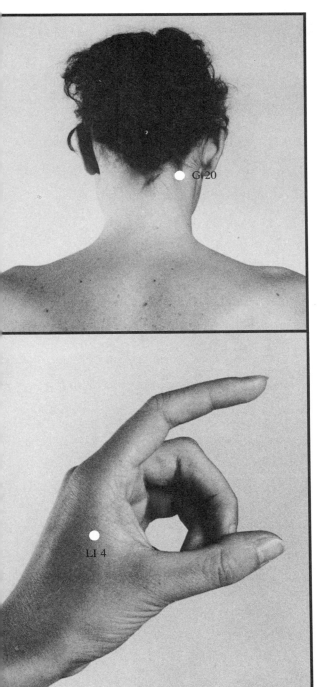

G 20 of the gall-bladder-meridian lies at the root of the hair on the outer side of the trapeze-muscle, where a hollow is easily felt when you move your head from side to side.

LI 4 of the large-intestine-meridian, called *Hegu,* "the enclosed valley," is on the metacarpus of the forefinger, on the top of a hillock that is formed by pressing the thumb against the side of the hand. Relax the hand before acupressing.

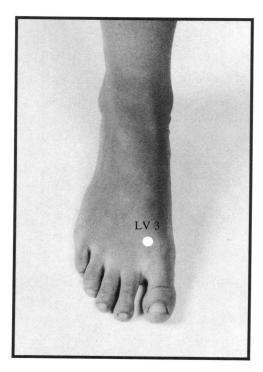

LV 3 of the liver-meridian, called
Taichong, ''flood-tide,'' lies two cun
away from the space between the
big toe and the second toe.

HIGH BLOOD PRESSURE

The blood pressure rises when the arteries are constricted and the circulation of the blood from the heart to the various parts of the anatomy becomes arduous. In elderly people calcification of the inner coat of the arteries often leads to arteriosclerotic high blood pressure. Indeed, in the past, high blood pressure seemed to concern almost exclusively elderly people. Nowadays the complaint is one that affects more and more people in their forties, in their fifties, even in their twenties. So there are other causes for high blood pressure beside calcification of the arteries. Stress and nervous tension can lead to constriction of the arteries as well.

There is nothing we can do for high blood pressure caused by arteriosclerosis, but if it is due to nerves we can do plenty, including fortifying the patient by means of acupressure. If you are already being treated for high blood pressure, you should always consult your physician first, since the blood pressure may react with some violence to stimulation by acupressing.

If the high blood pressure is due to stress, this stress is obviously the first thing to eliminate. It does not necessarily concern your environment. Being overweight frequently causes high blood pressure and the vessels have to cope with such a load that the symptom may well be considered to be one of genuine stress.

This brings us back to the A and O of Chinese medicine: a healthy, varied, reasonable and moderate diet. But do remember, if you are thinking of losing weight for the sake of your blood pressure, starvation or any other kind of drastic cure is about the worst service you can do yourself!

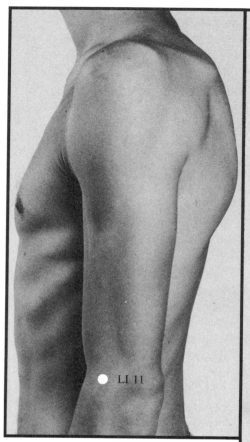

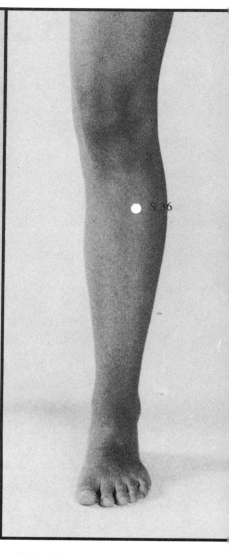

LI 11 of the large intestine-meridian, called *Quchi*, "the pool at the bend," lies at the end of the elbow flexor-fold, between it and the head of the humerus.

S 36 of the stomach-meridian lies three cun below the knee-cap down the shin and then one cun outwards on the same level.

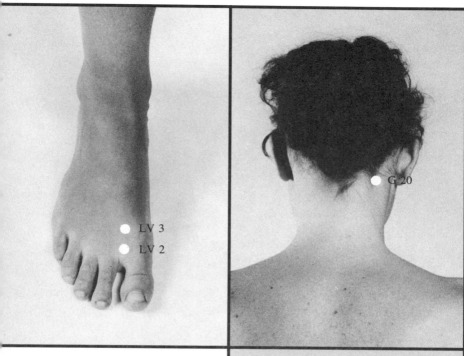

LV 3 of the liver-meridian lies two cun away from the space between the big toe and second toe, and LV 2 of the same meridian lies half a cun away from the same space.

G 20 of the gall-bladder-meridian, called *Fenchi*, "the windy pool," lies at the root of the hair on the outer side of the trapeze-muscle.

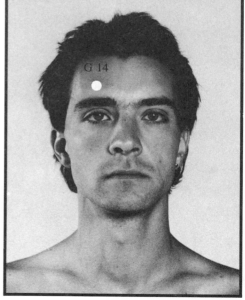

G 14 of the gall-bladder-meridian, called *Yanghai*, "the white Yang," lies one cun above the eyebrow, in a line with the pupil when you look straight ahead.

This is the way Dr. Hin sees the Oriental approach (top picture) and the Western approach (bottom picture) to Medicine. The sense of the Chinese text on the opposite page is as follows: "In the East, much care is taken to fortify the body, but not enough to combat the disease. In the West, the disease is dealt with most effectively, but not enough attention is paid to the body as a whole. The East attacks with an arrow, the West with artillery."

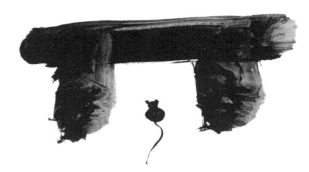

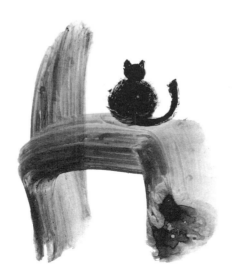

MEDICAL CO-OPERATION BETWEEN EAST AND WEST

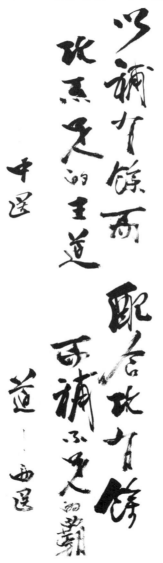

以補方藥而

比象天的主道

中醫

配合此有條

而補不足之

道·西醫

In the 1920's, at the time when Mao-Tse-Tung in China was calling for co-operation between Western medicine and the Chinese traditional School, the founders of the anthroposophic movement in Europe were anxious that contact should be established between different branches of medicine and the psychosomatic methods of therapy. This led to such developments as the modernization of homeopathy. The call for co-operation has already borne fruit. Acupuncture-anesthesia developed in China. There are hospitals in the Western world today where representatives of conventional medicine, homeopathists and acupuncteurs work side by side in close co-operation. Persons admitted for training in anthroposophic therapy must now have previously completed their medical studies in the State institutions.

However, much still remains to be done, and I do not think that the call for medical co-operation regardless of boundaries is any less urgent today than it was in the 'Twenties. Quite the opposite! Again, as when we were first discussing Inhoa and Chinese massage, let me remind you of *Kan*, the image of Water in *I Ging*, the Chinese book of wisdom: "Water reaches its goal by continuous flowing. It fills every hollow place before it flows on. Similarly, for the man of noble spirit, what is good must be rooted in nature and not appear only sporadically as if by chance. Also when teaching others, what matters is consistency. It is by repetition that the learner will assimilate the material."

Fields for Co-operation: Cancer and AIDS

What can these two diseases have in common for me to name them in the same breath? It is not their cause. AIDS is an infectious disease, propagated by the blood, sperm and excreta. The agent is a virus known as HIV. To be sure, cancer can be incited by a virus—it could be by HIV—but to date Cancer in man has not been found to be infectious and in the case of many tumors we still have no idea how the chaotic state of information within the cells and subsequent uncontrollable growth of neoplasm can have arisen. The manifestations of these two diseases likewise have little in common. There are too a great many different kinds of Cancer.

The factor common to both, which is immunity deficiency, is not obvious either. In AIDS the defense forces of the body are weakened by the agent itself, whereas in most cases of Cancer the immunity system suffers paradoxically from the therapy it receives. Radiation can touch the lymph vessels and cause permanent immunity deficiency. The cytostatica used in chemotherapy to date prevent the division of healthy cells as well as that of diseased ones. The patient, whether he suffers from AIDS or from Cancer, must be fortified and built up; in the case of AIDS, he must be able to survive chance infections and their therapy, in the case of Cancer, his body must resist the diseased cells and support chemotherapeutic cytostatica if his Cancer is to be kept at bay. Now, what can Chinese medicine do to assist?

Cancer

I am convinced that conventional medicine has already discovered the antidote for this disease. The weapons are there but we have not yet mastered their targetted, effective use. It is as though we had a new super-aircraft but no pilot able to fly it. As yet, chemotherapy has no selective preparations that attack exclusively the carcinogenous cells. So we have to protect the healthy cells from aggression as best we can. This is where our "gentle" medicine can prove useful, for we have natural curative means and acupuncture therapies that strengthen the immunity system and protect the healthy cells without fostering the diseased ones. A co-operation record highlights two main aspects:—Prior to and during chemotherapy, the patient's mind and body are fortified with the remedies of *gentle medicine* to help him to stand up to chemotherapeutical medication. His specific defenses against cancer are strengthened at the same time.—When the effects of the cytostatica become more than the patient can endure, chemotherapy is replaced by the methods of gentle medicine. Therapy combining acupuncture and mistletoe preparations has produced good results.

Attempts have been made in China to cure Cancer solely by the remedies of traditional medicine. These proved not to be strong enough to destroy the tumors, although the patient's defenses to resist them were considerably enhanced. The best results are obtained in China by means of a joint attack by Oriental and Western medicine working together and possibly in addition by the patient's utilisation of Chinese Yoga, Qi Gong, a suitable diet, and familiarity with Tao.

Aids

The factor AIDS underscores yet again the dual significance of prevention in the Chinese physician's understanding of the term: protection in health and protection in sickness. Man is born with his immunity system intact. Once his affectivity is perturbed and his body weakened, the system fails and he can no longer ward off infection. Stress, for instance, reduces physical immunity, independently of a person's age. Children too must be protected from stress and taught equanimity; they should be educated to use their faculties harmoniously and economically and shown how to fortify mind and body by an appropriate diet. Prevention in the first place is the protection of the healthy. Its other sense and objective, the protection of the sick, must be taken into account in the treatment of every ailment, whatever it may be. Every course of therapy must seek to cure the disease and to protect the patient from further aggression.

There is as yet no known cure for AIDS. Therefore prevention in every sense of the term is essential. Protection of the healthy is the purpose of the nation-wide campaigns that seek to promote "safe" intercourse by the use of preservatives and by refraining from hazardous sexual practises. The ancient Chinese rules of hygiene do not prescribe sexual abstinence but they advise economical utilization of the body-fluids. You must remember that for the Chinese any wound that bleeds is always something serious, for we see every drop of blood that flows away as a loss of our vital energy. Too much sex weakens the body. Protection of persons infected by the virus and therefore threatened by a multiplicity of complaints is a major concern for the AIDS Counselling Centers. The position is yet more critical when tumors or other chance infections have already set in. Such protection, in addition to that of the healthy, is the main objective of my own therapy. I am giving treatment, as an adjuvant to that of conventional medicine, to AIDS patients already stricken by the disease. HIV-positive persons who are not ill also come to me and ask for preventive treatment. It is in no-one's power to guarantee that these people will not fall sick. Chinese medicine can however fortify their mind and body and perhaps enable them to take better care of their health. For instance, if they want to give up smoking—a major health-hazard with or without AIDS—I can sustain their efforts with acupuncture. Alcohol, inappropriate diet, various factors of physical and mental stress that weaken the immunity-system, are things that we can discuss; some people do not seem to have the slightest idea of the extraordinary demands they are putting on themselves every day of their lives. Finally, I can show the people who consult me how to use the Inhoa method of self-massage, explaining its significance and advising them to make it a part of their daily routine. This enables them to fortify mind and body without outside help and not to lose confidence and self-assurance. I have noticed again and again that Inhoa helps people to shake off the feeling of being utterly forsaken that is usually the first reaction of those who have just heard that the results of their HIV-test were positive.

GLOSSARY

Acupuncture: The therapeutic insertion of needles at specific points of the anatomy called acupoints.

Acupressure: The therapeutic exertion of pressure on the same points as in acupuncture.

Adjuvant: An auxillary agent or remedy.

Anesthesia: Loss of feeling or sensation.

Auricular therapy: Treatment of the acupoints concentrated in the ear, which cover the same operational area as those disseminated over the anatomy.

Bioscopy: Examination of tissue taken from the living organism.

Cardiovascular: Pertaining to the heart and blood vessels.

Contraindication or counter-indication: A factor precluding the use of a given preparation or therapy.

Dietetics: The science of diet and nutrition.

Edema: An abnormal accumulation of fluid in intercellular spaces of the body.

Embolism: Vascular obstruction due to presence in the blood vessels of intravascular mass or a foreign body.

Emphysema: Abnormal presence of air or gas in body tissue.

Endoscopy: Endoscopic examination of hollow organs and body cavities by direct visual inspection.

Enteritis: Inflammation of the intestine.

Enuresis: Incontinence of urine during sleep.

Hemoptysis: The spitting of blood.

Indication: A factor pointing to the appropriate use of a given preparation or therapy.

Man: The male and female of the human species.

Moxibustion: The application of heat to the acupoints, largely by means of glowing artemisia-sticks, a therapy used in Chinese medicine together with acupuncture or acupressure.

Neuralgia: Pain in a nerve.

Physiology: The science concerned with the functions of parts and organs of living organisms.

Sciatica: Neuralgia and neuritis of the sciatic nerve, hip pains in acute or chronic form.

Sinusitis: Inflammation of the facial or cerebral sinuses.

Thrombosis: Formation of a blood clot within the heart or a blood vessel causing partial or complete occlusion.

Trigeminal Neuralgia: Acute pain in the trifacial nerve.

Urogenital: Pertaining to the urinary apparatus and the genitalia.

Yin and Yang: In Chinese philosophy, these are the two opposing principles of the universe. Primarily, Yin is darkness, Yang is light. Yin is the female principle, the Earth, all that is passive and flowing. Yang is the male principle, the Heavens, all that is active, energy. Yet Yang is present in every Yin, and Yin in every Yang. Man, the microcosm, is made up of Yin and Yang.